THE TRUTH ABOUT DISEASES

THE TRUTH ABOUT DISEASES

Causes, Precautions and Treatment - Without "Medicines" and Surgeries

TIHOMIR PETROV

author_{HOUSE}®

AuthorHouse™ UK Ltd.
1663 Liberty Drive
Bloomington, IN 47403 USA
www.authorhouse.co.uk
Phone: 0800.197.4150

Published by AuthorHouse 06/25/2014

ISBN: 978-1-4969-8485-2 (sc)
ISBN: 978-1-4969-8486-9 (e)

(Including incurable by the official medicine diseases: allergies, psoriasis, eczema, herpes, parodontitis, asthma, arteriosclerosis, gout, arthritis, disc disease, studs, nephritis, stones in the kidneys and in the gall bladder, ulcer, diabetes, hypoglycemia, tuberculosis, multiple sclerosis, cancer (tumors, cysts, myomas), AIDS, sinusitis, polyposis, mental illnesses, overweight, high and low blood pressure, migraine, anemia, osteoporosis, caries, leukemia, infertility, impotence, frigidity, menstrual problems or at a pregnancy, hepatitis, acute and chronic appendicitis, Parkinson's disease, dementia, enlarged prostate, epilepsy, cataract, glaucoma, etc..)

Contents

FOREWORD

Usually a man creates his diseases. In this book are explained the true causes for the diseases, principles of the Natural hygiene, which must be kept to prevent diseases and the way of treatment, if they have occurred. The Natural hygiene uses holistic/general way for treatment and maintenance of health.

They say that health is the greatest wealth. Usually we realize the value of something, when we lose it. Health is not everything, but everything without health is nothing!

Any theory is confirmed or rejected by practice. Think well what is true - theories that are taught in medical universities, which are not based on natural laws or the theories, based on natural laws and obvious facts!?

If the wrong/false theories, which are taught in the medical universities, that the causes for some diseases are "autoimmune", and other diseases are caused by viruses or bacteria, were true, most wild, free-animals in the Nature would also be suffering from the same diseases, from which suffer people. The truth is that very few of these animals get sick, and it is usually due to disposal of poisons in the Nature again by people.

The things are not so complicated as the "doctors" of the official medicine want to convince us. Otherwise, if there were at all live wild animals, most of them would also be ill, even if they had (veterinary) "doctors", "dentists", "doctors" of pharmacy and their poisons, called "medicines" and "vaccines".

We are creators of our tomorrow day and no need to pay to a "diviner", whether he is a doctor, a lawyer, a priest or a banker, to tell us what will happen to us tomorrow. Nothing special will happen. The inevitable will occur - we will reap what we have sown.

PART ONE

CAUSES FOR THE DISEASES

Few congenital diseases are hereditary. They are got due to genetic incompatibilities (close relationships, for example) or inherited by parents with disabilities. Most diseases are acquired and developed due to poor Natural hygiene, and mostly in poor inner purity of the body, i.e. due to poisoning of the body. The Natural hygiene means maintaining of good internal and external cleanliness of the body to prevent diseases. The body is self-purification, the self-healing and self-maintaining system. Another small part acquired diseases are developed because of lack of certain substances due to a systematic and prolonged malnutrition.

Four hundred years BC Hippocrates, the father of the medicine said: "Food to be your medicine and medicine - your food".

In 1862, Dr. Russell Thrall established in U.S.A. the "National Society for Hygiene", and in 1872 he published his work "A system of the hygiene". It preceded a number of books on Natural Hygiene, which emphasize the importance of diet for achieving and maintaining of good health.

In 1926 was published for first time the book "Toxemia explained" by the American physician Dr. John H. Tilden, in which he describes the cause for the diseases. After very thorough cogitations, observations, researches and experiments, he concluded that the cause for diseases was poisoning of the organism and especially poisoning of the blood (toxemia).

His theory, based on natural laws, repeatedly has been verified in practice and thus its correctness was proven. However, due to the extremely large financial interests of the official medicine and its political lobbies, there is censorship of certain informations and theories, while through the media are promulgated lies. Because of that the false theories and informations are not based on natural laws, illnesses and sick people, who believe of these theories, are increasing. Because of that the representatives of official medicine don't know the true cause for diseases or conceal it/played down, they continue to treat only the symptoms of diseases. And the truth is clear: when there is no cause, there isn't any consequence (in case - illness).

When in the body is accumulated bigger quantity of toxic substances than is released, it is obtained toxemia and a weakened immune system. The accumulation of poisons in the body occurs during direct ingestion of poisons, during the formation of waste products of metabolism, as and during deficiency of energy for neutralizing and excretion of toxins from the body. Metabolism involves two processes - anabolism and catabolism. During anabolism new body cells are built, and during catabolism sick, old and damaged body cells and waste cells from food are degraded.

Most waste products are formed from food, especially if it is not appropriate for an organism. Experimentally is found that most energy (up to 80%) is spent for digestion, and additional loss of nervous energy (during negative emotions - anger, fear) or energy spent for regulation of body temperature (especially in cold weather) reduces the body's ability to neutralize toxins and to release them. Poisoning of the organism causes disease (characterized by specific symptoms), which is toxic crisis - the body's attempt to neutralize and excrete toxins. During acute diseases, the action of poisons is relatively short, and after lowering the amount of toxins in the body below tolerance point, organism regaining his health. During chronic diseases, the action of poisons is long and/or frequently, thus damaging the tissues and organs, on which act poisons. For both the diseases location of impact of toxins usually defines the name of the disease.

Stress is a specific reaction (which is a specific symptom of a disease) of the body to any required adjustment or adaptation, caused by a harmful physical or emotional effect. It is carried out by a conventional method/way, based on the identical biochemical processes. In the physiological meaning, it is talked about stress, when it finishes with adjustment, i.e. without development of transient or persistent disease processes - that is called a "eustress". Stress, wherein is hampered the adaptation of the organism, as a result of which is developed a disease process, is called a "distress" (it is got due to poisoning of the body/blood).

To reduce the amount of toxins under the point of tolerance must: stop taking substances that act directly as a poison or their waste products are poisonous; to limit the loss of energy that is required and for neutralizing and releasing of accumulated toxins in the body.

"Lethal" and "pathogenic" microbes as "cause" for diseases.

Once almost all people thought and believed that the Earth was flat and that the Sun revolved around it. So and today for diseases most people still believe in myths, misconceptions and false theories, based on false assumptions and outright lies, which are supported by official medicine.

With development of the medical science through the centuries has been inculcated the modern faith in the established statement, inadmissible for discussion or doubt and accepted like unconditional truth, that diseases were caused by viruses or bacteria.

Initially it has been thought that the symptoms were diseases, with which must fight. The idea comes from the acient Greek philosopher Aristotle, who stated that any disease was determined by certain symptoms and it was the most important to give a name (usually - of the affected organ), i.e. to determine the diagnosis. This way of cogitation, which is the basis of modern medicine, justifies the widespread use of synthetic "medicines" and surgeries, which are unnecessary, damaging, disabling, and often causing and death.

During the last few centuries great importance for strengthen of the impact and prevalence of the transformed into dogma limited idea in the medicine has had the reductive perception of the French philosopher from XVII-th century Rene Descartes. He has argued that humans had two clear distinctive components: mind and specifically tangible physical body. According to him, the study of each one of them requires a separate methodology.

In support of the above perception in France has appeared the theory of the specific etiology, which has become one of the myths-pillars of the modern medicine. According to it, every disease is caused by a specific cause - such as a virus or bacterium. This theory is primarily a result of the discoveries of French chemist and biologist Louis Pasteur. Initially he had believed that the various "pathogenic" microorganisms caused diseases, and this has affected negatively on the development of the medical science, because it was accepted unquestioningly. According to him, there aren`t microbes in healthy tissues. But at the end of his life Pasteur questioned its basic views and before his death said: "However, the most important is the soil" – i.e. the state of the internal environment of the body and the strength of the immune protection are crucial to whether will be developed a disease. (This explains why very few wild, free-living animals in the Nature get ill, although they are not "immunized" with the poisonous vaccines and do not need (veterinary) doctors, dentists, pharmacists and their other poisons, called "medicines"!) Unfortunately, almost no one has taken into account his last words. Why? Because the official medicine is financially interested to there are sick people and new diseases.

Dr. Antoine Béchamel, bacteriologist and contemporary of Pasteur, has believed that microbes were an integral part of the living organism. According to him, microbes contribute to the process of digestion of food, waste products, sick and dead cells. The famous German bacteriologist Robert Koch shared the views of the Béchamel and also he has opposed to the theory of Louis Pasteur.

The great German scientist, father of the pathological anatomy - Prof. MD Rudolf Virchow, has said: "If I could live my life again, I would devote myself to prove that microbes seek their natural habitat - diseased tissue or decaying (fermenting) substances, and that they are not responsible for the development of any disease." And here are the words of Dr. George White:"If the microbial theory was based on real facts, there would not be any one living thing on the Earth!"

To prove the weakness of the theory of specific etiology, propagated by the supporters of Pasteur, Rudolf Virchow had drunk together with his students liquid, containing cholera vibrioes, but no one of them fell ill with cholera! Each one of us is convinced that, for example, during the "flu epidemic" there are many people who remain healthy, even though others around them sneeze, cough and "sprayed contagion". And why do only some people get sick? Because of toxemia and a weakened immune system.

Here is what Dr. John Tilden has written about microbes, such as "causes" for diseases: "In the beginning, when a man has begun to think what caused his indispositions, pains and diseases, he has done a monstrous mistake. He has decided that something beyond, outside of his desire brought the evil. The man, who is a religious animal, has thought from immemorial times that he has insulted with something one of his many gods. He still is burdened with centuries-old mythological heritage, which was taken out into white world after the theory for microbes, as a cause for the diseases, was "proven". It responded to his intuitive conviction for a demonic obsess about. After a long search, the man finally found "the demon - author" of all his woes. His efforts were rewarded, and remorse of his conscience for his past obvious transgressions - satisfactory excused. For 80 years, the "microbe-demon", doing evils, has been the explanation for the human mistakes, but these times were passing and mind was prevailing - the microbes were the last excuse, which people have invented to justify in front of the throne of their mind their mistakes, omissions and actions.

Microbes grow in a favorable environment - poisoned tissue by retained waste products, decaying or fermenting surroundings. Poor hygiene of the body - external and/or internal - creates these favorable conditions. These, who now preach fear from microbes are moral offspring of those, who in the past inspired fear from god, devil and hell."

You can read and two interviews **("The deception for the viruses" - the idea for "isolated viruses" – debunked /**by the link http://www.neue-medizin.com/lanka2.htm/ and **"No Panic. The Truth about bird flu (H5N1), vaccines and AIDS" /**by Google search**/)** with our contemporary Dr. Stefan Lanka - virologist and molecular biologist, who disproves the theory that diseases are caused by microbes.

PART TWO

Toxic (harmful) substances
for the human body

1. Foods. Experimentally is found that most energy is spent on digestion of food (up to 80%), absorption of nutrients, elimination and excretion of waste products from food. Much more energy is spent for the same processes, when food is unhealthy, unfit for an organism. And what foods are harmful to humans? First - all thermal-treated foods! Especially harmful are fried foods. They form strong acids and cause colitis, gastritis, ulcers, gout, arthritis, allergies, cellulite and lead to the formation of fatty plaques in blood vessels that cause high blood pressure, heart attack (infarct), brain hemorrhage, atherosclerosis, dementia and others. Also harmful are rancid, spoiled foods and GMOs. GMOs cause food allergy, increased toxicity, decreased nutritional value and others.

1.1. Mushrooms. It has been shown that in the mushrooms in the highest degree are accumulated radioactive substances, pesticides and harmful heavy metals - cadmium, lead, copper, mercury. Moreover, some species accumulate toxic substances, although they are from ecologically clean regions. These are for example field mushroom, sarnela, marasmius oreades, puffball and autumn vernal. Some bitter and pungent thrushes can be consumed only after boiling and the water must be poured. If they are not treated in this way, they cause pain and stomach/bowel disorders. The effect is due to containing in them toxic substances - terpenes, saponins and others, which are decomposed by heat treatment.

Mushrooms are rich in chitin, which overloads digestion. They also have a very large amount of fungal sugar (trehalose) and specific alcohol - mannitol. Trehalose is digested only by a specific enzyme. However, some people do not have it. In this case the fungal sugar ferments and causes severe digestive disorders. The mannitol causes high osmotic pressure in the intestines. Many edible mushrooms contain antibiotics, which can cause allergies. So that in some people after eating of non-poisonous mushrooms appear inexplicable at first sight symptoms of poisoning - nausea, pain, vomiting and diarrhea.

1.2. Animal products. Unfortunately for the gluttons, who want people to be omnivores or at least carnivores, it is not like that. Most people think, that they are omnivores: "But even our predecessors ate fruits, vegetables, nuts, seeds and meat, didn't they?" Every theory is confirmed or refuted by practice, and when the facts speak...

- After many studies and researches scientists have found that our ancient ancestors were also vegetarians. Only during the last glacial period, when it became impossible to feed with fruits, vegetables, seeds and nuts, to survive they began to kill animals, to eat them. Unfortunately, the habit to eat meat has existed and after the Ice era, because of necessity (for the Eskimos, the Inuits and other peoples who live far north and there is nowhere to obtain other food except meat - and therefore they live up to 50 years!), either by habit and/or suggestion of corrupt or ignorant "experts" ("doctors", "dietologists").

- Many scientific evidences prove that the consumption of animal products by humans, especially when it is frequent or prevalent, causes many diseases: asthma, arthritis, fever, tuberculosis, gastritis, colitis, ulcers, constipation, hemorrhoids, cancer, measles, osteoporosis, caries, tooth decay, purulent tonsillitis, gout, diphtheria, mumps, psoriasis, allergies, high blood pressure, heart attack (infarct), brain hemorrhage, atherosclerosis, sinusitis, obesity, migraine, cellulitis, etc..

- Anatomical and physiological characteristics of different types of animals and humans:

Carnivorous animals	Herbivores animals	Fruit eater animals	Humans
They have predatory claws.	They do not have predatory claws.	They do not have predatory claws.	They do not have predatory claws.
Lack of skin pores. Sweating by tongue for coolling of the body.	Sweating by millions of pores on the skin.	Sweating by millions of pores on the skin.	Sweating by millions of pores on the skin.
Cutting, long, sharp, conical (canine) fangs for tearing of meat.	Front teeth like incisors to tear the grass, and rear - molars by which they grind food.	Front teeth like incisors for biting of food, and rear - molars through which grind food.	Front teeth like incisors for biting of food, and rear - molars through which grind food.
Their jaws can only move up and down to grab and tear.	Their jaws can move and sideways, to be able to grind food.	Their jaws can move and sideways, to be able to grind food.	Their jaws can move and sideways, to be able to grind food.
Small salivary glands in the mouth.	Well developed salivary glands in the mouth.	Well developed salivary glands in the mouth.	Well developed salivary glands in the mouth.
Acid saliva, required for degradation of proteins. It does not contain the enzyme ptialin.	Alkaline saliva containing enzyme ptialin, required for pre-digestion of carbohydrates.	Alkaline saliva containing enzyme ptialin required for pre-digestion of carbohydrates.	Alkaline saliva containing enzyme ptialin required for pre-digestion of carbohydrates.
Stomach, producing from 10 to 20 times stronger hydrochloric acid for digestion of animal proteins.	Stomach, producing from 10 to 20 times weaker hydrochloric acid.	Stomach, producing from 10 to 20 times weaker hydrochloric acid.	Stomach, producing from 10 to 20 times weaker hydrochloric acid.
Intestines are only 3 times longer than the body, so that it can be more quickly disposed rapidly putrescent / decomposing/ proteins and their highly toxic waste products.	Intestinal tract, 10 times longer than the length of the body. Plant food does not spoil (not rot) so fast, so it can pass slowly through the body, making possible to extract everything valuable from it.	Intestinal tract, equal to 12 times body length. Fruits do not rot (not spoil) so quickly, so they can pass slowly through the body, making possible to extract everything valuable from them.	Intestinal tract, equal to 12 times body length. Fruits vegetables and nuts do not spoil so fast, so that they can pass slowly through the body, making possible to extract everything valuable from them.
The liver can eliminate 10 to 15 times more of highly poisonous uric acid (a waste product of animal proteins).	Liver does not produce the enzyme urikaza and can eliminate the minimum quantity of highly toxic uric acid.	Liver does not produce the enzyme urikaza and can eliminate the minimum quantity of highly toxic uric acid.	Liver does not produce the enzyme urikaza and can eliminate the minimum quantity of highly toxic uric acid.

From which it follows that people are fruiteaters!

- The healthiest and longest-living people are vegetarians! They feed with fruits, vegetables, grains and nuts, as prevails raw food, which is its natural state. "Vegetarian" comes from the Latin word "vegetus", which means "strong, healthy."

1.2.1. Meat and meat products.

For information of the ignorant, who "competent" state that "fish and chicken flesh is not a meat" (and maybe according to them fishes and birds are plants, and not animals!), it is also a meat, but with different content and structure. All heterotrophic organisms (those that feed with ready organic substances), with the exception of micro-organisms and mushrooms, i.e. all animals have flesh (meat).

Perhaps the most frequently asked question, related to nutrition, health and weight loss (slimming) is: "What is the way to get the necessary proteins?" Proteins are the most complex nutrients. They are degraded and absorbed the most difficultly, and to them for these processes is consumed most energy. If animal proteins are properly combined, they pass through the whole digestive tract of humans for more than 24 hours! Actually, we don't need so much quantity of proteins as "experts" want to make us to believe, nor they are more important than carbohydrates or fats, for example. First, the body recycles 70% of the protein wastes. Second, the body loses only 23 g proteins daily. It becomes by urine, feces, sweat, falling hair, scaling of skin.

The meat is declared for the most ideal source of proteins for humans, because the human proteins look more like animal proteins than vegetable. By this logic, it is best to eat even a human instead of animal meat! The truth is that the specific proteins of an organism are not received directly by consumption of protein food. The proteins from food first are degraded to amino acids, and then body builds its necessary and intrinsic proteins. To what extent the specific proteins are produced from food, depends on how the amino acids are used from it. People, as fruiteating animals degrade easier and faster plant proteins, and thus it makes better use of amino acids from vegetable rather than animal products. All the nutrients are absorbed the most complete, when food is in its natural state, i.e. raw. Amino acids are very sensitive. From the high temperature of cooking many of them are destroyed or coagulate, so that the body can not use them. They become poisonous, lead to weight gain, create unnecessary work of the body and thus it results in a loss of energy. In other words, to be meat less harmful to humans and therefore more amino acids to be used, it should be consumed raw as predators eat it. Meat also contains a large proportion concentrated fats. Not such, which donate energy, and such which causing heart attack (infarct) and brain hemorrhage. During thermal treating, especially during frying, occur irreversible biochemical reactions, which form fatty plaques that accumulate in blood vessels. After some time, when blood vessels are constricted enough, are got atherosclerosis, heart attack (infarct) or brain hemorrhage. The situation accelerates and worsens if by one or another reason is formed thrombus.

All nutrients are created in the plant kingdom. There are 23 different amino acids. 15 of them are built in the body of animals and humans. The other eight are called "essential" or "indispensable" ("vital") and can be obtained only from plants. All raw fruits and vegetables contain most of them, and some of them (carrots, bananas, cabbage, maze/corn, cucumbers, eggplants, peas, potatoes, squash, tomatoes) contain all of them. Nuts, sunflower, sesame, peanuts, and legumes also contain all eight amino acids. If you regularly eat raw fruits, vegetables and nuts, you will receive all necessary substances, including amino acids. In emergency situations, when the body is unable to provide the necessary amino acids, it gets them from their amino acid stores. And when the body has an excess of amino acids, it stores them in the same stores.

Another argument, which is emphasized in favor of meat is that it gives us power. The most important requirement for a food is it to fill up the body with fuel, and that to be used for production of energy. For fuel are used carbohydrates, and factual the meat does not contain any. In fact the fats, which are contained in meat, are converted to carbohydrates, but this is with limited effectiveness and continuous process, which occurs only when the body's reserves of carbohydrates are exhausted. Furthermore, usually meat is consumed by humans heat-treated, which makes it much more difficult-degraded, difficult-assimilated, and also it forms fatty plaques and strong acids. It should be clear that fats in the body are accumulated not only by fats from food. The excess carbohydrates in the body are converted into fats and stored as a reserve. Fatty deposits can be considered as "carbohydrate banks" in which, if necessary, is "invest" and "withdraw".

At low amounts of hemoglobin (anemia), doctors recommend eating of foods with animal origin (especially meat), because there the concentration of iron (an essential element for building of hemoglobin) is biggest. (Hemoglobin is a iron-containing pigment in red blood cells /RBCs/, whose primary function in the body is the transport of oxygen and carbon dioxide.) But this is only true for raw animal products, because after heat treatment is destroyed and most of the iron in them! But even if they are eaten raw, they are sufficiently harmful to human body. From foods that are suitable for people most iron contain raw leafy vegetables, beet and beans.

Finally let us mention vitamin B_{12}. The theme about this vitamin is part of the myth for irreplaceable of animal proteins. It is said, that if a man does not eat meat, body will experience a shortage of vitamin B_{12}. (Poor herbivorous animals! How do they get this, if they do not eat meat? Or they do not need it?) This is nonsense. Like the other "arguments" of "experts", that it is vital to eat meat! How do the fruiteating and herbivorous animals /to which we belong, due to our anatomical and physiological characteristics/ obtain vitamin B_{12})? It contains in small quantities in plants. But mainly it is produced in the human body. In stomach is produced a substance, called "intrinsic factor", which carries the produced by the bacterial flora in the guts vitamin B_{12}. Our actual needs of vitamin B_{12} is negligible. One milligram of vitamin B_{12} is enough for two years. A healthy person has a reserve for five years. But here is where the trap - decaying hampers of the secretion of so-called "intrinsic factor" in the stomach and slows the production of vitamin B_{12}. This fact was known and was discussed in a report, titled "Vitamins of B group", appeared in the yearbook of the Ministry of Agriculture of the United States in 1959. And propaganda states just the opposite! Therefore, more the carnivorous than the vegetarians experiencing a shortage of vitamin B_{12}. On the one hand, as the meat is usually consumed heat-treated, all the vitamins and enzymes are destroyed (and other substances and micro-elements are virtually unusable), and from another - because of the strong acid and rotting meat - is disordered acid-base balance in the body. Then there are other troubles - constipation, gastritis, colitis, ulcers, gout, arthritis, colon cancer, etc..

For rapid increasing of growth and weight to most animals are given hormones, which by meat, milk and eggs are deposited in people, thereby they can disrupt their hormonal balance. (This is one of the causes for abnormal or degenerated people - gays, homosexuals, transvestites, lesbians. Other causes are: vaccines, narcotics, "medicines"). In addition of that, to animals are given "medicines", such as penicillin, tetracycline, arsenic and others to "protect" against diseases or for "treatment". By fodder in animal may enter pesticides, radioactive elements, herbicides, etc.. You might say, that plants are treated also with chemical fertilizers, but the concentration in meat is much greater, because to obtain 1 kg of meat, an animal eats much more plant food. Furthermore, the meat is treated with sodium sulphate, to mitigate the smell of decay and to impart a pink color instead of gray tinge of carrion (dead flesh).

1.2.2. Eggs. Somebody may have heard, that eggs were very useful, because they contained high quality proteins. We do not need such, and easily digested amino acids. The eggs, as animal proteins, even if they are raw, are very hard degradable (as are formed harmful waste products) and hard absorbable into the human body. And if they are heat-treated, due to biochemical reactions, coagulated proteins and amino acids will become more difficult-degradable. See the difference between raw and cooked yolks and whites. Eggs contain and many lipids.

1.2.3. Milk and dairy products. The best and only adequate food, but only for babies of mammals is fresh and raw milk of the relevant mammal! Only the people (except of some animals to which people give milk) after being weaned, continue to drink milk and eat dairy products.

Usually people consume milk and dairy products from cow milk. Enzymes, necessary to degrade milk are renin and lactase. In most mammals (humans are also mammals) they are ceased to be produced, after they are weaned. In humans - after completing of the third year. In all milks is contained the ingredient casein, that is difficult degradable. In cow's milk, which is most often used by people, the casein is 300 times more than in human milk! The casein is used for building of bones. Even if the cow milk is raw, it coagulates in the stomach and forms large, tough, dense and hard-degradable secretions, in the form of clots (such as cooked egg white), which are suitable for four-stomach digestive tract of the calves. The human body spends much quantity of energy for digestion, absorption of some of the milk, neutralizing and disposing of harmful waste products from it.

The things get much worse, because milk and milk products normally are consumed heat-treated. They are at least pasteurized. Pasteurization was invented by the French chemist and biologist Louis Pasteur, once he had done the wrong assumption, that microbes were the causes for diseases. During pasteurization, food is being heated to 72 degrees Celsius for at least 15 seconds or up to 138 degrees Celsius for at least 2 seconds, as the purpose is to be destroyed the "pathogenic microbes". Above 50 degrees Celsius are destroyed all vitamins and enzymes, and biochemical processes, which are taking place, make other substances in food unabsorbed or hard-absorbed. Part of the milk solidifies, builds up along the inner walls of the intestines and prevents the absorption of nutrients from the body. The result is sluggish bowels. In addition the by-products from the degradation of milk, emit very toxic mucus in the body. It is highly acidic and part of it is stored, so that later it can be further processed.

Exactly that mucus is the cause of rhinitis, sinusitis, (bronchitis) pneumonia, pleurisy, meningitis, migraine, skin allergies, psoriasis, purulent tonsillitis, earache, etc.. And the acids cause osteoporosis, gastritis, colitis, ulcers, gout, arthritis, thyroid problems, etc..

Some believe that dairy products are very useful, because of calcium that they contain. Ignorant or well-bribed "experts" have taught us (and continue to lie us), that if we did not consume dairy products would be sick of osteoporosis (porous bones) or caries (tooth decay). The teeth and all our other bones will become fragile. But data show, that just the biggest consumers of dairy products most suffer from caries and osteoporosis, and also from other diseases. As already it was mentioned the cow milk, which was the most widely used by people, was intended solely for feeding of calves until they were weaned! First - even if the milk is raw and is consumed by human babies, who still suck milk and still they have the enzymes renin and lactase, needed for digestion of milk, it remains very difficult degradable, as casein in it is 300 times more than in human one. Second - one of the main functions, for which is used calcium in the body, is to neutralize acids. All animal products, except butter, even crude are highly acidifying. The organism draws calcium from its stocks, to produce calcium carbonate compounds, with which to neutralize received acids. True irony is that people eat dairy products, due to calcium into them, and the available calcium in the body is taken to be neutralized the acids from the same dairy products.

In fact all leafy green vegetables contain calcium. All raw nuts too. The raw sesame seeds contain more calcium than any other food on the Earth. Most fruits also contain calcium in abundance. If every day you eat enough raw, fresh fruits and vegetables, and two or three times a week half a cup of raw nuts, you can never experience a shortage of this element (if you do not overdo acid forming substances).

Moreover, for savings in dairy products often are added cheap and harmful hydrogenated and hydrolyzed vegetable fats (see for details in the section on margarine and sodium glutamate).

1.3. White flour.

Everything, which is mentioned for white refined sugar, goes for white flour and dough products made from it. Eat wholegrain wheat bread. Unlike white flour, in the wholegrain flour remain the germ and the brans of the grains. They contain many valuable vitamins, enzymes, microelements. Moreover the brans help for peristalsis of the bowels.

1.4. Soya.

Soya has been used mainly as feed for livestock, for production of margarine, fats for sweets and snacks, soy sauces. And in industry – for manufacture of plastics, fibers, paints, etc.. Lately, it is recommended as a substitute of meat, milk and products from them. It is advertised as a "perfect food".

The advance in technologies make it possible to produce isolated soy protein from that, which was formerly considered as waste product - the defatted residues of pods with high content of proteins, which look and smell awful. But thanks to the numerous artificial colours, flavors, stabilizers, preservatives and others, this disgusting product becomes a pleasantly redolent and delicious "food."

In fact, soya contains many harmful substances. First of them are potent enzyme inhibitors, that block the action of trypsin and other enzymes, needed for degradation of proteins. These inhibitors are not completely degraded by heat treatment. They can cause serious gastrointestinal complaints and chronic amino acids deficiency. If soya dominates in menu, it may occur a damage/harm to the pancreas. Because the quantities of carbohydrates and proteins in soyabeans are almost equal, alkaline and acidic stomach juices, which are released for their degradation, are neutralized, and food ferments, begins to rot and gases are produced.

Soya also contains hemagglutinin, which generally contributes to blood clotting, and therefore can form dangerous clots in blood vessels. Hemagglutinin and the enzyme inhibitors of trypsin suppress growth.

Soya contains substances, that suppress thyroid function.

Soya is one of the plants, that contain the highest percentage of phytic acid. It blocks in digestive tract absorption of zinc, calcium, magnesium, iron and copper.

Isoflavones (these are phytoestrogens - substances with a structure similar to the female hormone estrogen) that are present in soya in large quantities, especially genistein and daidzein, are toxic. During researches is found, that they suppress the synthesis of estradiol and other steroid hormones. Therefore, soya and soya products, but from time to time and in limited quantities are useful for menopausal women or those who have problems with estrogen balance. However, children and men in general do not need these substances at all! As a consequence of abuse with soya and soya products can disrupt hormonal balance and to obtain early maturation of girls and change the sexual orientation of boys.

Another argument, that breast milk is best for babies, and not to substitute with soya milk, for example - it was found that soya milk has 10 times more aluminum, and at the same time lack cholesterol, lactose and galactose, which are necessary for the development of the nervous and skeletal systems.

1.5. Margarine.

It is promoted as a healthy substitute of cow butter. The truth is that it is cheaper, but extremely harmful for health. It is obtained from cheap, inferior vegetable oils (including soya), which by **hydrogenation** process become solid at room temperature and much more durable product than butter. During hydrogenation are being added hydrogen atoms to molecules of double bonds of unsaturated fatty acids (contained primarily in vegetable oils) to become saturated. High pressure, temperatures from 120 to 210 degrees Celsius and the presence of metal catalysts, such as aluminum and nickel, are required so this process to be carried out. Moreover, all the vitamins, enzymes and microelements are destroyed, and large part of the fatty acids, that normally exist in the so-called "cis-configuration", pass into unnatural transformation. In the finished product there are also residues of metal catalysts, which are highly toxic to the body.

As in the Nature there are only natural "cis-", but not of transformed fatty acids, the human body can not cope with their digestion and absorption, they begin to accumulate into cell membranes (in some of them quantity is up to 20%, and should be zero!) and on other places, where must not be at all (fatty plaques in blood vessels). This violates the protective functions of cell membranes, cell nutrition and metabolism, as a whole. The presence in the body of unnatural trans-fatty acids and lack of essential fatty acids leads to cardiovascular diseases, allergies and other diseases. Trans-fatty acids prevent the conversion of cholesterol in the body. The quantity of low density lipoproteins (LDL) is increased - an important factor for the development of atherosclerosis, heart attack (infarct), brain hemorrhage and others, and at the same time is decreased the quantity of high density lipoproteins (HDL), which protect the cardiovascular system from the first ones.

Trans-fatty acids increase the amount of prostaglandins E2 (hormones that enhance inflammatory reactions), while suppress the formation of prostaglandins E1 and E3, which have anti-inflammatory effect. Prostaglandins regulate many processes, involved in metabolism, and their impaired balance leads to allergies, problems with coagulation, formation of fatty plaques in blood vessels, etc..

The type of the dietary fats, which are taken, affects to the composition of the cell membrane, and hence to the proper operation of functions into the cell. Dietary fats act as solvents and carriers of fat-soluble vitamins A, D, E, and K, and they are the only provider of polyunsaturated essential fatty acids - EFAs. Taking enough of them is very important for proper function of the immune system. EFAs can not be synthesized by the body, and only can be got from food. They are two main types – omega-3 and omega-6 fatty acids. EFAs are contained mostly in the following foods, which are suitable for people: cold pressed oils of flaxseed, rapeseed, sunflower, in wheat germ, raw nuts. EFAs are easily destroyed by heat treatment and in contact with air.

EFAs are necessary for building of healthy cell membranes. They help for lower cholesterol, protect against the development of cardiovascular diseases and are a major precursor for the formation of prostaglandins in the body. Also they participate in the transfer of oxygen from the air into the lungs through alveolar membranes to hemoglobin in the blood, and then through the cell membranes - to mitochondria.

Finally - in any case do not eat margarine. From time to time may be consumed little butter, coated on a slice of bread.

1.6. Chocolate.

The chocolate contains a number of harmful substances: sugar or artificial sweeteners, milk, hydrolyzed and hydrogenated oils. But even the pure chocolate (the **cocoa**) contains theobromine - harmful substance, which is similar to caffeine. Several researches show, that the theobromine is cancer-generating. Moreover it causes atrophy of testises.

2. Spices (seasonings, condiments).

2.1. Salt.

The word salt comes from the Latin word "sal". In the past salt was called "white gold". It was a cause for political fights and wars. The Roman soldiers were paid with salt, from which derives the word "salary" (wage). Salt was very valuable to people and was exchanged for gold with the same weight.

The Egyptians used salt for embalming of the Pharaohs. It is good to remember that! It is still used for preserving of food products, because it kills all microorganisms and prevents dead products to ferment and decompose. But the salt dries and kills all living cells!

Salt consists of 95% sodium chloride, the rest being impurities such as iodine, iodine stabilizers (such as glucose), aluminum silicate, which prevents the salt from absorbtion of moisture (but it is highly toxic to the nervous system) and many others. Salt is obtained in salt mines and then refined, as most of the minerals are removed until remains only sodium chloride, which is just a white poison. When sodium chloride is mixed with water, regardless of whether before to enter into the body or after that, are formed sodium hydroxide and hydrogen chloride. Sodium hydroxide has a highly corrosive action, and chlorine was used as a chemical combat substance during World War I.

Salt as and other toxic products cause thirst and water retention in the body. This is a protective function, by which the body dilutes received poisons. Our body is able to eliminate by the kidneys a maximum of 1.3 to 2 grams of salt per day. Our organism recognizes table salt as an aggressive cellular poison, an unnatural impurity and wants to eliminate it as quickly as possible, to protect itself. This causes overworking of the organs, which are involved in the release. The kidneys are most overworked. They can be seriously harmed and to be got nephritis. Salt damages the nervous system.

The causes for constantly high blood pressure are narrowed blood vessels by fatty plaques, polluted kidneys or use of narcotics. Salt is one of the biggest polluters of the kidneys. Because the body cannot eliminate excess sodium chloride, the organism tries to isolate it. In this process water molecules surround the sodium chloride and neutralize it. For this process the cells consume perfectly structured cell water, to neutralize sodium chloride. This causes dehydration of the cells and their death. If the quantity of sodium chloride is still high, recrystallization occurs of the excess salt, as the body uses non-biodegradable proteins and produces uric acid. It is very poisonous to the body and to neutralize, it is connected with sodium chloride. New crystals are formed, which are deposited directly into the bones, joints, blood vessels and organs. This is the reason for rheumatism, arthritis, gout, stones in the kidneys and the gall. Recrystallization is a natural body protection process, but if this situation persists, the body is poisoned by these substances. Dehydration of cells leads to cellulite and dehydration of the body.

Myth is the need to take salt tablets during hot weather. Some "experts" argue, that during profuse sweating and loss of water are being lost and valuable minerals. According to the real results of scientific researches have been found, that after the first few days of acclimatization people stop to lose salt by sweating. Salt only contains sodium, chlorine and sometimes artificially added iodine. Sodium and iodine, and all other microelements, vitamins, enzymes, etc., people can get by eating of enough fresh, raw fruits, vegetables and nuts. Chlorine, as already was mentioned, is a poisonous chemical element, so it is better to be avoided.

Instead of the poisonous cooking salt for seasoning can be used crushed sea salt. It is usually considered as crude salt and it is extracted from the ocean or the sea by evaporation. Usually manufacturers do not refine it, so it contains traces of other minerals, including iron, magnesium, calcium, potassium, manganese, zinc, iodine and others. To use it, however we must be sure that it has not been subjected to refining. Natural sea salt is a healthy substitute of the cooking salt and contains over 80 minerals, necessary to maintain the body's cells, but better use no more than 2 grams per day!

2.2. White refined sugar.

White refined sugar contains only what scientists call "empty" calories, i.e. pure, refined carbohydrates. In plants there are not pure sugars - nature has combined them with vitamins and micro elements, which are necessary and sufficient to ensure their digestion and absorption by the body. And as in the process of refining of sugar cane and sugar beet vitamins and micro elements are extracted or destroyed, to digest and absorb the resulting unnatural refined product, the body begins to draw from its reserves of enzymes, proteins, vitamins, sodium, potassium, magnesium and calcium. The last one is extracted from the bones, thus they become porous and brittle. The intake of calcium tablets can not compensate the loss of this mineral, because it is absorbed in a very low quantity, and furthermore it overworks the kidneys and liver and can accumulate in some tissues and organs.

Calcium is essential for the regulation of acid-base balance in the body. In 14 point scale 0 means totally acidic, 7 - neutral, and 14 - all alkaline. The healthy human blood is slightly alkaline and pH must be in the range between 7.35 and 7.40. The intake of sugar and sugar products induces the formation of strong acids. To neutralize them, body extracts calcium from bones, which is necessary for the production of alkaline compounds. This leads to caries, cavities and porous bones.

Under the influence of refined sugar is reduced the secretion of gastric juices and is slowed peristalsis of the stomach. Sugar enters quickly into blood, where its quantity increases much (hyperglycemia). The aim of the hormone insulin, secreted by the pancreas, is to reduce high blood sugar level. But in some people that level is decreased rapidly and below normal, and it is got hypoglycemia, which is with some of the symptoms: dizziness, weakness, sweating, anxiety, insomnia, etc.. In that situation, the adrenal glands are activated and they mobilize reserves of glycogen in the body. It is degraded to glucose, to restore the normal blood sugar level. Thus, may occur diabetes (permanent hyperglycemia) or hypoglycemia, depending on that which gland is exhausted faster - pancreas or adrenal. Numerous experiments have demonstrated clearly, that sugar leads to depletion of micro element chromium from the body, which is most important for the absorption of insulin and for maintaining of glucose metabolism.

The body converts the sugar and in form of reserve polysaccharide glycogen is stored in the liver. The possibilities in this respect are limited and excess sugars are further converted into fatty acids, which are accumulated into the subcutaneous fatty landfills. Normal human weight is calculated as follows: from the height (in cm) is subtracted 100 and the difference is reduced by 10%. At overweight of 20% over the norm, begins deposition of fatty tissue and around internal organs. For example, around blood vessels, heart and kidneys, and this leads to a violation of their functions. The intake of refined sugar increases blood cholesterol.

Sugar makes kids hyperactive and nervous, because it is a very potent stimulant for the adrenal glands. Consumption of it can increase the level of the hormone adrenaline up to 4 times, which is a typical stress response of the organism. The result is increased production of cholesterol and hormone cortisone, which suppresses the immune system.

Sugar has very adverse effects to the brain and nervous system. When its refining is incomplete, toxic metabolites are received, which hinder of oxidation processes in nerve cells. Significant intake of sugar and sugar products causes, by forming acids, destruction of beneficial bacteria that produce B vitamins necessary for proper functioning of the central nervous system. Consumption of such refined products leads to a preponderance of the exciting processes in the cerebral cortex and the appearance of vegetative dystonia - a very common diagnosis. White refined sugar, sugar products, white flour and all products should be totally excluded from the menu for people with mental illnesses.

All artificial foods, artificial drinks, food additives, preservatives, stabilizers, emulsifiers, artificial flavors and artificial colours (abbreviations "E with numbers") are harmful for living organisms!

2.3. Saccharin (E954).

Saccharin is artificial sweetener. Its main ingredient and trivial name is benzoic sulfimide. It is a low energy substance and is 300 times sweeter than sucrose (sugar), but it is with unpleasant taste. After its consumption remains bitter-metallic taste, especially at high concentrations. Saccharin is unstable, when is heated and does not react chemically with other food ingredients. Mixtures of saccharin with other sweeteners are used to compensate of weaknesses and shortcomings of each sweetener. Proportion 10:1 (cyclamate: saccharin) is a frequent combination in countries, where these sweeteners are legal. In this combination, each of these sweetener masks the taste of other. Saccharin is often used together with aspartame. Saccharin is the oldest artificial sweetener, produced in 1878 by chemist Constantin Fahlberg. Strongly was enhanced its use during World War I, when there were enormous shortages of sugar.

It became even more famous and fashionable between 1960-1970 year, when mass it began to be recommended by nutritionists with a primary quality, as a good sweetener with no calories. In the United States saccharin is known as "Sweet'N Low", distributed in little pink packages.

In 1989, after many laboratory tests, the Office of Environmental and Health Hazard Assessment (OEHHA) in California, stated saccharin as a carcinogenic chemical. Officially it is prohibited to be used in many countries. And in countries, where it is permitted for use, the packages must be labeled with "Harmful for health".

2.4. Cyclamate (E952).

It is 30 times sweeter than sugar and is used to neutralize the bitter taste of saccharin. It is a carcinogen and is prohibited in many countries, including the United States. It is not recommended for pregnant women, children and people with kidney diseases.

2.5. Aspartame (E951).

Aspartame (Nutra Sweet, Spoonful and Equal measure are different trade names in English) is an intense sweetener, approximately 200 times sweeter than sugar. Despite of its approval in the U.S. and its presenting as a "safe" additive, aspartame is one of the most dangerous substances, produced ever for the unsuspecting public and it is the most dangerous supplement for foods, beverages and "medicines". It has been used worldwide in soft drinks and other low-calorie or sugar-free foods since 1974 till today.

According to official statistics since 1985 in the U.S. have been made over 10 000 reports about side effects after use of aspartame. (In the best case the reports are 10% of all cases! It means, that the actual number is at least 100 000!). Aspartame causes headache/migraine, dizziness, fainting, nausea, muscle spasms, weight gain, rashes, depression, fatigue, irritability, tachycardia, vision problems, breathing difficulties, mental anxiety, dizziness, tinnitus, memory loss, joint pain and others., as have been reported and even death cases!

Also, as per observations by independent doctors and scientists, the use of aspartame can cause or complicate the following diseases: brain tumors, multiple sclerosis, epilepsy, Parkinson's disease, Alzheimer's disease, birth defects, diabetes, chronic fatigue syndrome, syndrome of deficiency attention, autism and others.

Aspartame consists of: aspartic acid - 40%, phenylalanine - 50%, methanol - 10%.

Aspartic acid. The free aspartic acid is a cause of many acute and chronic effects, because it and her compound "aspartate" belong to the so-called "exci(ting)-toxins" (stimulants, exciters). Usually these are amino acids that interact with specific receptors in the brain. Too much quantity from this amino acid can increase the levels of aspartate in blood plasma, which enters into the brain and slowly destroys neurons. Up to 75% of these neurons can be damaged before to occur clinical symptoms. In some people/age groups, the risk is greater, because the areas of the brain are not fully protected by phisical barriers.

Aspartame and glutamate, in general are normal existing neurotransmitters in the brain, which carry out the transmitting of information from one nerve cell to another. But when their levels are increasing, it leads to death of neurons, due to the entering of much calcium in them. That is why these compounds belong to the exciting toxins, because they stimulate too much the nerve cells and cause their destruction. Blood-brain barrier, which is composed of specialized capillary structures and normally protects the brain from excessive inflow of exciting toxins, is not fully developed in babies, children and sick old people. In them this barrier may omit these substances in the brain.

In diabetics, for example, it happens very often and aspartame can lead very quickly to memory loss and confusion. According to diabetologist Dr. Hyman Roberts from the American Diabetes Association, aspartame leads to the occurrence or worsening of diabetic complications, such as retinopathy, cataracts, neuropathy and gastroparesis. It also causes seizures (insulin reactions), complicated absorption by diabetics of insulin or oral medications. Major improvements have been noted in the functions of the sick people after avoiding of aspartame and rapid complications, when a patient starts again to take aspartame. The use of aspartame in hypoglycemia is more dangerous, because it can cause disorientation, dizziness or epileptic seizures.

Aspartame changes the level and of neurotransmitter dopamine, and accordingly deteriorates condition of people suffering from Parkinson's disease.

The exciting toxins can cause and death, because one of the main areas in which they operate is the hypothalamus (part of the brain), which in turn can cause sudden heart rhythm disturbances and myocardial infarction.

Phenylalanine is an amino acid, which normally is found in the brain. Intake of aspartame, however, increases in undesirable quantities its presence there, especially if it is combined with high carbohydrate consumption. People, who cannot well degrade and absorb phenylalanine, and for them foods, which contain Nutra Sweet are even more dangerous.

This can lead to very high, sometimes even fatal concentrations of this amino acid in the brain. At the same time it is occurring decreasing of the amount of serotonin (another brain neurotransmitter), causing depression, major mood swings, anger, etc..

Methanol (methyl or wood alcohol) is very powerful poison, that causes damage to the optic nerve and irreversible blindness, as and can lead to death. The permitted maximum amount of methanol per day was 7.8 mg. And one liter soft drink, sweetened by Nutra Sweet contains at least 56 mg of methanol!

Methanol is gradually released in the small intestine, when aspartame meets enzyme chymotrypsin. This absorption is increased, when aspartame is heated above 30 ° C, and this is temperature in human body. At this temperature is monitored and the breakdown of methanol to formic acid and formaldehyde. During the "Desert Storm" in Iraq the american soldiers cooled themselves by large quantities of sweetened drinks with aspartame. The same soldiers now are suffering from diseases, similar of formaldehyde intoxication.

In addition to the serious vision problems, some other symptoms that are caused by methyl alcohol are headache, ringing and buzzing in the ears, nausea, gastrointestinal disturbances, weakness, neuritis, etc..

The methanol from aspartame enters very quickly into the bloodstream, further is degraded to formaldehyde, which in turn is oxidized to formic acid. Formaldehyde is highly neuro-toxic compound, allergen, mutagen, teratogen and carcinogen. For information, formalin, in which are preserved biological tissues and carcasses, is a 30-40% solution of formaldehyde. Formaldehyde is a main raw material in industry for obtaining of insecticides, dyes, explosives, adhesives, etc.. Formic acid is used in industry and for removing of paint, because is highly corrosive.

Researches in recent years show that during consumption of aspartame is increased the level of formaldehyde in all tissues and organs, as it leads to permanent and irreversible harms. This breakdown product is highly toxic for proteins and DNA, as it causes and genetic defects. Some people need very small doses, to appear harms.

Burning in the mouth, which is being felt during the consumption of products, containing Nutra Sweet, is due to formaldehyde, which burns the tongue and creates a bitter taste.

The manufacturer of aspartame (the company "Monsanto") uses various arguments to prove "harmlessness" of the product. One is that in some fruits and vegetables also there are phenylalanine, aspartic acid and methanol. But there these compounds do not exist in free form, as they are in aspartame, and they are connected with balancing and antidotes amino-acids.

Diketopiperazine (DKP) is a compound, that is produced in significant quantities during the breakdown of phenylalanine in soft drinks during prolonged storage. When it enters into the guts micro-organisms produce nitrosated compound, which is similar to the chemical substance N-nitrosourea, a powerful cause of tumors. There are ample evidences from researches, showing that aspartame causes cancer in the brain, uterus, ovaries, testes, breast and pituitary. Unfortunately, many of the researches and their results have not seen light of day. Today also deliberately is hidden information about the brand Nutrasweet. From 1973 to 1990, as the product was not stopped, the occurrence of brain tumors in people over 65 has increased to 67%.

Aspartame causes addictive (stronger than that to alcohol), especially if are consumed more foods and beverages, in which it is contained.

2.6. Acesulfame K (E950) /Sunette, Sweet one/, which is 200 times sweeter than sugar, has not affirmed its reputation yet. It is used most often in combination with aspartame - the first gives momentary sweetness, and the second - the sensation of sweetness afterward. It is known, that it can cause allergies, tumors in the lungs, mammary glands, thymus gland, thyroid, leukemia, etc..

2.7. Cyclamate. Artificial sweetener, that is carcinogenic.

2.8. Sodium glutamate. It is met as mono sodium glutamate (MSG) or accent. It is another exciting toxin, which is widely used in food industry to provide an additional taste of food. It consists of about 78% glutamic acid (glutamate) and 22% sodium.

Glutamate, sold as a spice, is in free state. Unlike that, in the algae it is connected with other compounds and antidotes - this is the substantial difference! Researches show that tomatoes and mushrooms contain very little amount of free glutamic acid, but that has nothing common with highly concentrated product, for example as hydrolyzed vegetable protein.

During the last four decades were collected enough evidences, that mono sodium glutamate in the free state is a health hazard. When eating foods that contain glutamate as a condiment, may be experienced the following symptoms and health effects: numbness, tingling and chest tightness, palpitations, weakness, insomnia, headaches, cramps and abdominal pain, visual changes, serious damages of retinal, lesions (damages) in the brain, neuro-endocrine disturbances, destruction of nerve cells in the hypothalamus, obesity, etc.. Glutamate is especially dangerous for babies and children, because they are still with immature blood-brain barrier and through it can more easily pass toxic substances.

Glutamate is normally existing and even is the most common neurotransmitter in the brain, but its concentrations are negligible. When its quantity is increased, the activity of neurons is harmed, and at higher concentrations neurons die - analogous to aspartame. Exactly the free aspartate and glutamate are toxic, and not connected, which are found in the natural foods. The connected glutamate is degraded more slowly and in this way it is absorbed more slowly, so that it can be utilized by the body, and excess quantity - eliminated, before to reach a toxic concentration.

Blood-brain barrier, that obstructs toxins to reach the brain cells, is designed in the case to protect the brain from occasional increases of glutamate up to moderate grade, which could occur after the consumption of certain foods. But it is not intended to eliminate high concentrations of glutamate and aspartate, which are consumed daily with artificial foods and drinks. Moreover, in brain there are some areas, where this defense system does not work - hypothalamus, pineal gland, area

THE TRUTH ABOUT DISEASES

postrema. The most important from the listed is hypothalamus, as it is the neuroendocrine control center, associated with sleep, emotions, regulation of the immune system and the autonomic nervous system. The Increased levels of glutamate into the blood can easily increase and those into the hypothalamus. Repeatedly has been proven destructive effect of mono sodium glutamate to a small, but very important control area in the hypothalamus, called "nucleus arcuatus".

Another way of disposing of excess glutamate is by its connecting in brain with certain molecules, which transport it to the appropriate nervous cells. But due to the constantly high affluent of exciting toxins, this system is also limited at some time. The exciting toxins cause generation of free radicals, which on the one hand directly damage/harm neurons, and on the other hand - in the process of lipid peroxidation is being released a substance, that obstructs of the molecules, transporting of glutamate, which leads to its accumulation into the brain. When free radicals are being produced, the first place, where damage occurs, are cell membranes, which are composed of molecules of polyunsaturated fatty acids, and they are very susceptible to such attacks. This process of oxidation of membrane lipids is called "lipid peroxidation" and is provoked by hydroxyl radicals. Similar processes occur not only in brain, but also in other organs and tissues in the body. This contributes to the development of disease processes. It is known that degenerative diseases of the nervous system are associated with its damage/harm by free radicals.

In most cases the processes evolve gradually, slowly and insidiously, as just in sensitive people are developed quick reactions. Glutamate and aspartame can cause or worsen **Alzheimer's disease, Parkinson's, multiple sclerosis, ALS, etc.. Amyotrophic lateral sclerosis (ALS, sometimes called Lou Gehrig disease, Charcot's disease or disease of the motor neurons)** is a progressive, almost invariably fatal disease. ALS is a neurological disorder, which is characterized by progressive degeneration of motor neurons - cells in the spinal cord and main brain, causing paralysis and death. ALS subsequently leads to atrophy of muscles and the brain loses completely its ability to control them. Several researches have shown that people with ALS had significant accumulation of products of lipid peroxidation in the spine, as a result of interactions with free radicals, including iron.

Perhaps many doctors do not know that the free iron is one of the most serious sources of free radicals. And also it is very often advertised by the medical industry and is often added to many foods, beverages, sauces, spices, do not to mention for vitamin formulas, in which they present continuously.

There is MSG in hydrolyzed vegetable protein, hydrolyzed oat flour, sodium caseinate, calcium caseinate, soups, etc.. The **hydrolyzed products** are usually derived from plants with high levels of glutamate. First they are boiled for several hours in containers with hydrochloric acid. Then, to neutralize the last one, is added caustic soda (sodium hydroxide) - one of the strongest bases, which burns tissue paper, leather, etc.. The resulting slurry on surface is harvested and dried to become powder. It is with high content of exciting toxins and various carcinogens. Then to it is added and pure mono sodium glutamate. This toxic mixture then is added to various "foods" - such as in soya products, malt extract, broths, various flavorings and spices.

Other powerful exciting toxins are L-cysteine and homocysteine. High levels of homocysteine are determined as a major indicator for heart diseases and brain hemorrhage.

2.9. Hot/chilli and sour.
Hot chilli foods and spices, especially strong chilli, such as chilli paprikas, black pepper in powder, white pepper in powder, red chilli pepper in powder and others, as and concentrated acids (vinegar, pickles etc.) and acid forming foods, are extremely harmful for the body. According to some "experts" the hot chilli is useful in gastritis, colitis, ulcers and other diseases, because it kills "pathogenic" bacteria! If you have already read and realized that germs are not causes for diseases, you wouldl easily find the real reason and for these diseases. Inflammations and wounds on the skin and mucous membranes are caused by mechanical and/or chemical irritations! Exactly the hot chilli, concentrated acids and acid forming foods cause chemical irritation and primary mucosal

inflammation (gastritis, colitis), and then wound (ulcer). And the bacteria in the stomach and intestines actually are useful. They help for digestion of the food and the waste products, as and for absorption of the nutrients from them. Salt also produces strong chemical irritationof mucous membranes.

3. Narcotics.

All narcotics (including informally stated for narcotics, such as cigarettes, alcohol, coffee, not herbal tea, "medicines"), are highly poisonous for the body.

Using of narcotics is like playing with fire - always there are risks. Among the risks are: the danger of physical and/or psychological dependence; tendency to aggression, hypomania, depression and suicide.

The effect of a narcotic depends very much on the state and mood of the user, at the time, when the substance is taken. Many narcotics exaggerate this mood and may have effects that are different from those, expected by the user. A dissatisfaction can turn into a deep melancholy, an anxiety can turn into panic. A narcotic may not be well received by the body and to lead to nausea, vomiting and sickness.

The use of narcotics is especially dangerous for people, who are psychologically vulnerable, people with diseases of heart, kidney, liver, lungs and other, people with mental health problems and pregnant women. Women, who breastfeed should be aware that they can deliver the active ingredient of the narcotic to the baby by the milk, which it drinks.

With the use of certain substances there is a risk of overdose or lethal amounts of consumption. Some users deliberately intake a high dose. Most often what happens is, that it is consumed something other than, what the user expects to be accepted. These are cases, when a pill or powder does not contain, what the seller has declared. There isn`t quality control for the illegal narcotics. Users can also take both narcotics with different effects that are often unpredictable and sometimes fatal.

Narcotics affect to the perception of reality and the user's ability to concentrate. In city traffic or at work the use of narcotics may increase the potential for accidents. The use of narcotics while driving is punishable by law. As a result of use of narcotics can worsen performance in school and at work.

Risks, associated with use of narcotics depend and on ways of usage. "Infectious" diseases like AIDS and hepatitis are actually caused by poisoning of the body and reducing of the protective functions. Sooner or later the narcotics like all other poisons, damage/harm kidneys, liver, lungs, brain and other organs, as and the immune system as a whole.

Officially stated for narcotics are the illegal: cocaine, heroin, cannabis (marijuana, hashish, anja, joint, indian hemp, trumps, cac, kif, Marie Jeanna, pot), kratom, LSD, peyote, salvia, magic mushrooms, Hawaiian rose, amphetamines (cathinone, mephedrone), methamphetamines, ecstasy (MDMA, MDE, MDA, MBDB, MDEA); legal components of the so-called "medicines"- (DMT, DXM, GHB, mCPP, PCP, ketamine), opiates (morphine, codeine, tebain, papaverine, noskapin, methadone), "benzodiazepines" (sleeping pills, tranquilizers), antidepressants and psychostimulants; anabolic steroids (anabolic androgenic steroids / AAS /, "steroids").

Unofficially stated for narcotics, legally and most widely used are: alcohol, tobacco and other tobacco products, coffee, not herbal tea, Coca cola, Pepsi cola and others, that contain caffeine, so-called "medicines".

3.1. Alcohol. For some people and minimal quantity of alcohol is dangerous/harmful: pregnant and nursing women, as and those who are trying to become pregnant; dependant from narcotics; people, in whose families there are cases of alcoholism; people, taking different "medicines"; people suffering from certain diseases and people who drive or operate machines. Use of alcohol poses risks that are greater, when it is drunk in excessive quantities at a single occasion, when it is drunk systematic even of small quantities or when quantities are increased regularly over time.

Drinking of alcohol in very large quantities in a short time can lead to unconsciousness, vomiting and death from asphyxiation. In even larger amounts of alcohol, it can cause alcohol poisoning, coma and death.

The alcohol often leads to incidents that may threaten life and health of the user and others. For example, in falling, driving or operating machines.

Women, who drink during pregnancy may have children, who suffer from abstinence syndrome or who have severe defects of the face, decreased brain weight and delayed mental and physical development. These birth defects, called "fetal alcohol syndrome", are incurable.

The alcohol can be very dangerous, when is used in combination with other narcotics and "medicines". The combination may lead to death due to:

- heart failure (due to overstretch of the heart muscle or stopping of the heart due to delay in breathing);
- liver failure (it occurs, when the body is unable to eliminate alcohol and other narcotics/"medicines", because of that occur poisoning and stopping of the work and of other organs);
- cessation of breathing (it occurs, when the lungs stop to work, due to taken quantities of depressants of the central nervous system; such "medicines"/narcotics suppress center of breathing in the brain, so it slows down until it stops).

Long-term and excessive use of alcohol can lead to the development of tolerance, physical and psychological dependence. People with developed physical dependence suffer from abstinence symptoms when trying to stop drinking (eg, tremors, sweating, anxiety, insomnia, delirium). The presence of abstinence symptoms is one of the criteria for diagnosing of alcohol dependence. Alcohol is also acid-forming.

Alcohol causes and many purely physical disabilities and diseases, some of which are:

- brain damage/harm, leading to Korsakov syndrome (alcoholic dementia);
- premature aging of the skin;
- cancer of the throat or mouth;
- weakened immune system;
- weakening of the heart muscle, which can lead to heart attack (infarct);

- high blood pressure and brain hemorrhage;
- anemia and abnormal blood clotting;
- breast cancer;
- damage/harm to the liver - cirrhosis, cancer;
- kidney damage/harm;
- lack of vitamins, leading to various diseases;
- bleeding (especially in advanced cirrhosis);
- severe inflammation of the stomach (gastritis), ulcers, cancer;
- polyneuropathy (damage/harm to nerves of whole peripheral nervous system);
- obesity or malnutrition;
- gout, arthritis, osteoporosis and caries/tooth decay - because alcohol is highly acidifying;
- diabetes, due to damage/harm of the pancreas.

3.2. Cigarettes and other tobacco products.

More than 4 000 substances are contained in tobacco smoke. Many of them are toxic, others are radioactive, and over 40 cause cancer. The reason for this is the high temperature (up to 900 degrees Celsius), which is being developed in the smoldering end of the cigarette during a inhalation. About 85% of tobacco smoke in a confined compartment is due to indirect stream smoke. It contains 2 times more nicotine, 5 times more carbon monoxide, 3 times more the carcinogen benzopirene.

Nicotine - the main reason for creating psychological and physical dependence. Through the lungs and blood vessels nicotine reaches the brain in 7 seconds of ignition of a cigarette. It leads to increasing of the rate of blood stream due to constriction of blood vessels and increasing of blood pressure values.

Tar - oil combination of 60 substances that cause cancer. It damages/harms lung tissue. It stains fingers and teeth.

Carbon Monoxide - it pushes the oxygen from red blood cells, resulting in the tissues, and especially heart receive less oxygen. Carbon monoxide is a highly poisonous gas.

Cadmium - blocks the action of an important element of growth - zinc. This leads to a delay in the development of the child, who is born underweight.

Smoking can cause:

• ischemic heart disease and heart stroke;
• chronic obstructive pulmonary disease (asthma);
• cancer of the lung, mouth, throat, bladder, kidney, pancreas, esophagus, stomach, liver, cancer of the blood;
• disease of the blood vessels of the lower limbs (Buerger's disease);
• brain stroke;
• aortic aneurysm;
• pneumonia;
• cataracts;
• impairment of the function of the reproductive system;
• damage/harm to the fetus.

Women who smoke during pregnancy are at high risk for developing osteoporosis, cardiovascular diseases, chronic bronchitis and emphysema, cancers. More severe course of pregnancy is caused by smoking. The unborn child also becomes a "smoker."

Risks for pregnant women:

• increased risk to the fetus;
• premature birth;
• stillbirth;
• death of the child immediately after birth;
• birth of children with disabilities;
• lower birth weight babies.

Although the insoluble tars are a contributing factor to become ill from lung cancer, the real danger is radioactivity. According to Everette Koop, (former Secretary of Health of the U.S. government) radioactivity, but not tar is cause for at least 90% of all cases of lung cancer, associated with smoking. Tobacco is fertilized with phosphates, rich of radium 226. In addition, many soils have naturally high levels of radium 226.

Radium 226 breaks down into two components with long life - lead 210 and polonium 210. These radioactive elements are extracted from the soil and pass to the fibers of tobacco leaves.

The researches show that lead 210 and polonium 210 deposits are accumulated in the bodies of people, exposed to cigarette smoke. Data from 1970 show that smokers have three times more of these elements into the lower lungs than nonsmokers. In smokers also is found a greater accumulation of lead 210 and polonium 210 in their skeletons, though there are not studies that link these deposits with bone cancer. Polonium 210 is the only component of cigarette smoke, which produces tumors by itself after inhalation during experiments with animals. When a smoker inhales cigarette smoke, the lungs react by forming irritated areas in the bronchi. Any smoke causes this effect.

Although these irritated spots are considered as potential tumor damages/harms, they are completely natural defense system and usually disappear without harmful effects. Insoluble tars in tobacco smoke can slow this healing process by adhering to lesions and causing additional irritation. In addition, tobacco smoke causes the bronchi to constrict for long periods of time, which obstructs of the lungs to get rid of these residues. Polonium 210 and lead 210 in tobacco smoke tend to accumulate on the branches of the bronchi. When smoking is continued for long periods of time, deposits of radioactive elements turn into radioactive 'hot spots' and remain at bifurcations for years. Polonium 210 radiates alpha radiation, for which is proved that causes cancer. As the polonium 210 has a half-life of 21.5 years, it could jeopardize the ex-smoker after years, since the smoking has been stopped. Experiments, measuring the level of polonium 210 in victims of lung cancer, have found that the level of "hot spots" was the same in smokers and former smokers, even when ex-smokers had quit five years before their death.

More than half of the radioactive materials, emitted by a burning of a cigarette, are released into the air where they can be inhaled by non smokers.

It has been also proved that tobacco smoke can contribute to airborne radioactive particles to collect in the lungs of both smokers and non-smokers, exposed to second hand smoke. Studies on uranium miners, which had showed an increased risk of lung cancer due to exposure to radon, have been repeated in smokers again, to measure the risk of lung cancer from radioactive radon in indoor air. It turns out that tobacco smoke plays role of a kind of 'magnet' for airborne radioactive particles, causing them to accumulate in the lungs, instead on furnitures. (Smoking in enclosed places greatly enhanced risk of lung cancer.)

It is estimated that the total accumulated quantity of alpha-radiation from smoker to his 60 years of age, who has used a pack of cigarettes per day in a confined space is from 38 to 97 rad. (Two packs a day bring to 143 rad, and in non-smokers take no more than 17 rad.) Exposing of 1 rad per year yields a 1% risk of lung cancer (according to the lowest estimations.)

Nicotine, the active ingredient in tobacco smoke, has been known for long time with its high level of addiction. In fact, doctors and pharmacologists haven't reached to consensus about the question, which causes more addictive - nicotine or heroin. Physical dependence occurs, when a chemical becomes essential for the body or for functions of metabolism. In other words, when for a substance is said that causes physical addictive, it is understood that its prolonged use makes in the body tolerance to the extent, that at discontinuing use causes adverse side effects. Called "abstinence symptoms", they can include anxiety, stress, trauma, depression or physical conditions, such as shakes or nausea. It would be better to avoid these consequences, as you do not use substances that cause them.

Nicotine is also a toxin (it can be fatal, if it is intaken in large quantities). It is proved that nicotine has an adverse effect on the heart and circulatory system, causing a constriction of the veins and arteries, rapid pulse and high blood pressure, which in turn can lead to fainting, brain hemorrhage or heart attack (infarct). Nicotine damages/harms the blood vessels most commonly of the legs, it can cause **Byurger's disease** - gangrene (decay), which is most often in the lower extremities, which requires amputation. In fact nicotine is so poisonous that smokers, who ignore the advices, given by their doctors, and continue to smoke while using patches to quit smoking, manage to overdose themselves and die from a heart attack (infarct) or brain hemorrhage.

The disturbing thing about all this information is that most people still are unaware of the radioactive risk from cigarettes. In fact many physicians, scientists and health administrators, either have never heard about polonium 210 or consider it just for another terrible story. Why is this information so hard to be perceived? When studies first appeared in the late 1970^{-s}, many magazines were unable to print articles, because their main advertisers, companies producing cigarettes, threatened that they would pull their money, if they published the facts. Although network news picked up the story, virtually nothing came out in print. Those, who had heard the information, were hard pressed to show collaborating evidences and ultimately were convinced that there was nothing to worry about.

The power of the tobacco industry to suppress information goes far beyond magazines. Tobacco lobby in Congress has provided subsidies for decades and has fought against the laws that could harm the American tobacco industry. Tobacco interests practically possess Senate, as many campaign subsidies come exactly from the cigarette profits. The money from the tobacco business also go and to fund organizations, such as the Partnership For A Narcotic Free America, which accepts a sharp agenda against narcotics, but it does not include alcohol and tobacco as narcotics yet (claiming they are harmless). For example, in 1984 was passed a law that aimed tobacco manufacturers to provide a public list of substances that caused dependence, which were used in the manufacture of cigarettes. This list is now in the Department of Health and Human Services, with the stipulation, that it can not be shown to anyone else.

In the past many companies have been known that they have added chemicals to cigarettes for flavor, as many of them have maintained a level of dependence. In Britain such chemicals contain acetone, turpentine and other substances, about which are known that are carcinogenic.

Tobacco companies argue, that revealing their "secret ingredients" will decrease their competitiveness. In fact, when in Canada was passed a law, forcing the list with additives to be available to everybody, one large company corrected recipe for cigarettes, which have been imported into Canada, and another one took its product out of the country entirely.

Smoking also leads to skin aging, hair loss, impotence, etc.. Carcinogens, which are contained in tobacco smoke, penetrate into the blood through the lungs and thus they poison the body.

3.3. Caffeine.

Caffeine, intaken in normal dosages (about 100 mg) increases resistance to muscle fatigue. It narrows blood vessels in the brain and therefore it is contained in many "medicines" against headache, but widens the blood vessels in the rest of the body. Caffeine increases heart rate and blood pressure.

The way that methylxanthines (in particular caffeine) affect to the brain, has not been fully investigated yet. Most likely they block brain receptors for the neurotransmitter adenosine - a substance that is synthesized in the brain, regulates the processes of sleep and inhibits physical activity. It seems that caffeine exerts its stimulatory effect by inducing of release of catecholamines (and especially of norepinephrine) - substances, also produced in the brain, which increase physical energy and excitement.

It is generally believed, that caffeine significantly stimulates intellectual ability and it actually increases sensory sensitivity and mood, but its stimulant action refers mostly to the increased performance on a physical level, especially when one is tired. Undoubtedly, the caffeine causes insomnia and as such it is superior to any similar means, as its intake does not affect to the normal course of sleep, when a man sleeps after the disappearance of its effect.

In 70^{-s} of XXth century by researches was proved that prolonged use even of small quantities of caffeine can cause unpleasant effects such as insomnia, palpitations, arrhythmia, anxiety, and the chronic abuse leads to so-called "caffeine intoxication".

The caffeine intoxication is characterized by worry, anxiety, insomnia, palpitations, gastrointestinal problems and mood changes. Treatment of caffeine intoxication includes reduction and stopping of use of foods and beverages, containing caffeine.

A cup of coffee or another drink, containing caffeine, passes through the kidneys and urinary system for 24 hours and overburdens the kidneys very much. In this case isn't it better to drink decaffeinated coffee? Usually caffeine is extracted chemically, using highly corrosive chemical solvent, which remains in the grains and must be neutralized and disposed from the body. But even if the decaffeination is made by steam, the coffee remains strong acid forming, which is big enough problem for the body. The acids slow down digestion, causing fermentation and putrefaction of food. In addition, increased acidity in the blood causes water retention in the body and/or extracting of calcium from the teeth and other bones to form carbonates, which are necessary to neutralize these acids. Acids also irritate the mucous membranes of the stomach and intestines.

Other narcotic drinks, containing caffeine are black and others. types non-herbal tea, Coca cola, Pepsi cola, Red Bull, Pit Bull, etc..

Decaffeinated non-alcoholic beverages are sufficiently harmful to the body, because of their content of phosphoric acid, sugar or artificial sweeteners, colourings, stabilizers and preservatives. In general, soft drinks are highly acidifying, i.e. poisonous to the body.

Physically exhausted organs are recovered only by rest. A tired brain from lack of sleep becomes stupid and can be restored only by sleeping!

3.4. "Medicines".

There aren't medicines! The "medicines" are what people want. The "medicines" are what the "doctors"-pharmacists pretend that create for treatment, but the only thing, which they have achieved is a relief. Besides the representatives of the official medicine, which earn for the expense of health and life of ignorant patients from production and sales of poisonous "medicines", which are useless and at the same time are harmful, earn and self-appointed quacks-"healers": homeopaths, herbalists, extrasensory, needle-therapists, masseurs, "seers", etc.. Whatever therapy and/or "medicine" to use and apply, they only suppress symptoms, as they can not eliminate the cause of the disease. Herbs and "medicines" on herbal base, as and disgusting looking and even more disgusting stinking ointments in their best case can bring temporary relief.

These, who look for medicines outside themselves, they look for them in the paradise of fools. Worse than the folly somebody to buy a "medicine" is he to remain so ignorant that to believe in the healing power of the "medicines". The periodicity, which characterizes all the functional abnormalities in the body only supports the assertions of proponents of the "medicines", that they have been cured by them. And the truth is that the disease has taken its normal course - the poisons have decreased below the point of tolerance despite the "medicines", and not because of them. The only "positive" thing, that is achieved by so-called "medicines", is suppression of the symptoms of a disease, such as removal of the pain or stopping of the excretion of toxic waste products (different secretions). Just stopping of neutralizing and disposal of toxins from the body is one of the damages/harms, which cause the "medicines".

Stopping or delaying of the excretion of toxins from the body actually slows treatment. On the other hand, the direct or indirect damages/harms of the kidneys, liver, brain, immune system, and hence the body as a whole are some of the side effects, for which are blame the "medicines". All "medicines" - from the first to the last - are poisonous. The effects of the minimum, "safe" doses, for which the representatives of official medicine claim, that are harmless, occur over time. "Drop by drop - a reservoir is formed." Especially during prolonged, frequent or systematic use of "medicines". By the way - "antibiotic" literally means "against life"! And in fact, antibiotics destroy not only the "pathogenic" microorganisms, but also leukocytes /white blood cells/ - defenders of the organism /antibodies/ and all living cells indiscriminately!

Why do the "medicines" harm and kill? Pharmaceutical companies manage to impose their "cures" by briberies, false advertisements and different ways for circumvent of the laws of different countries. Most disturbing is the fact that by counterfeit and adjusted "safety tests" they often present dangerous substances ("medicaments") for harmless and even useful. The manipulation is done in several ways. First, by frauds during the clinical tests. Companies can easily require (by bribery) to be made relevant to their interests researches, which could help for patenting of their products ("medicines", vaccines, anabolics, supplements - vitamins, minerals, etc.). The incentives and temptations for the people, who make experiments are large. At least 1 000 USD average are paid for testing of one person, so some doctors can even get to 1 million USD per year for testing of a new medicine! These doctors know that if they do not provide such data as are expected from a pharmaceutical company (and not as they are in fact), in the future can not rely on subsidies or income from the firm. The situation is similar and in animal experiments.

There are different ways to falsify data from a study:

- it is not reported for died or refused patients at the time of clinical tests;
- modification or replacement of the results;
- presentation of false results, supported by reputable physicians;
- providing of a political lobby;
- conflict of interests.

In general, pharmaceutical companies don't pour millions into the vaults of political parties, and give money to some individual politician or public figure among those, who set health policy. Serving to themselves with the help of a congressman, they receive very favorable market conditions that provide them long-term gains. As the documents disclose the pharmaceutical industry buys legislation and legalizes its crimes.

The experiments with animals (vivisection) are the best-developed form of organized, officially acknowledged cruelty over animals. It is supported by the most lucrative industries and multinational corporations. Huntingdon Life Sciences (HLS), for example, is the largest working under a contract laboratory for animal tests in Europe. Every day there are killed about 500 animals during the testing of pesticides (and other chemical fertilizers), colourants, preservatives, flavorings, household cleaners, "medicines", vaccines etc.. In their laboratories usually there are about 70 000 animals - rabbits, cats, dogs, guinea pigs, mices, birds and primates. These animals are doomed to die in cruel sufferings during the "humane" experiments.

As the animals more or less differ anatomically and physiologically from the humans (the most similar to us are the monkeys), the adverse effects (if we may say that there are some useful), in particular of the "medicines" to humans are unpredictable. From which it follows that the cruelties during experiments on animals are not justified. Here's the opinion of one of the world-renowned toxicologists - Prof. Gerhard Zbinden from the Institute of Toxicology in Zurich: "Most adverse reactions of acute or chronic toxicity, which occur in man, can not be demonstrated, anticipated or avoided by the usual experiments with animals.... Most experts think the modern, routine toxicological procedures for fruitless endeavors, during which the scientific ingenuity, creativity and common sense are replaced with mindless filling of standard protocols." Dr. E. Marshall from Baltimore writes: "Even when a "medicine" has undergone a complete and an adequate pharmacological test to several animal species and has been found to be relatively nontoxic, subsequently often has been found that it could cause unexpected toxic reactions of sick people. This has been known since the birth of scientific pharmacology!".

Many substances, which are highly poisonous for humans are safe for different animals. We know, for example, that arsenic can kill a person, but is also safe for guinea pigs, chickens and monkeys. Green fly agaric, which has caused the deaths of many people was harmless for rabbits. The botulinum toxin that kills a mouse and a man, can not harm to the cat. The antibiotic chloramphenicol can cause harm to bone marrow of humans, but not of animals.

If the "medicines" are tested according to the actual requirements, the vast majority of them should not be marketed, because of their harmfulness and ineffectiveness. And of course many pharmaceutical companies would bankrupt. Dr. Herbert Gundeshaymer explains: "The results from experiments with animals are not comparable between species, and therefore can not guarantee the safety of people.... In fact the purpose of these tests is not to protect the consumer from unsafe products, and these corporations from legal liability." When people are harmed as a result of a "medicine" and if they try to take legal actions against the manufacturer, then it can justified that the legal tests for safety have been adhered, and so it is exempted from liability for the blame for putting of a dangerous product on the market. Although there are reliable and accurate scientific methods for evaluation of the toxicity and efficacy of new "medicines", such as: in vitro cultures, chromatography and mass-spectrometry, quantum pharmacology, properly conducted clinical experiments etc, they are not applied, because the results will not cover the requirements for safety and effectiveness.

Conflict of interest means that the experts, participating in relevant committees for approval of "medicines", are dependent and/or they have some financial interests in companies, whose products will be tested. In other words, either they themselves have participated in developing of the product, or they have been sponsored by the companies to carry out seminars, or to give "consultations" in relation to it, or directly have been bribed for its approval.

During clinical experiments with humans must be fulfilled certain conditions, which are hard achievable in developed countries. The patients must be informed for the risks during testing of a medicament, to know the indications for use of it, to have information for alternative therapies and that they can cede during the experiment. All this is confirmed with a voluntarily signing of an informed consent. Also the duration of the tests and the number of patients, on which medicaments are tested, are greater.

So that tests are preferred to be made in developing countries, where and costs are much lower. Legislation in these countries is not so strictly and there is less bureaucracy. Moreover, in poor countries there are more often certain diseases. People there agree easier, because they need medical care and often lack the financial resources for that, and also there are more illiterate and less educated, which make them easier to be more easily persuaded or deluded to participate in experiments. Doctors in these countries also are susceptible to financial inducements, which pharmaceutical companies offer them to raise a number of patients on who to test a new "medicine", which is not approved yet in some developed country.

Artificial vitamins and nutritional supplements are also harmful, because they harm too much kidneys and liver, and also they are not absorbed so well as natural ones.

4. Vaccines. "When once somebody intervenes in the order of the Nature, no one knows how will end all this." All vaccines are poisonous, because they contain various substances, which are harmful for health and are at least allergenic for the body: traces of antibiotics, aluminum salts, thiomersal (mercury derivative), formaldehyde, etc.. Vaccines are produced by infection with the corresponding virus of cell cultures of monkey, dog and bovine kidneys, chicken embryo, human aborted fetuses and others, which are rich of foreign for the human body proteins and DNA. Their aim is to create immunity in the body. Could this become by making a mild form of measles or other similar disease by poisoning of the body with pathological products?! Only a deformed thinking can reach to such a conclusion!

Vaccines and autogenic "medicines" are made from products of the disease and the idea that they create immunity against a disease is the final product of such a ill thinking. (The same goes for the "medicines" - diseases are "treated" with poisons, and the same diseases are caused by poisoning of the body!) The truth is, that the diseases, against which are used vaccines, have decreased significantly before to start mass immunizations by improving the hygiene and nutrition of the people. By vaccines just is checked the status of the immune system, and if the quantity of toxins in the body is enough to be suppressed the strength of the organism, an additional poison, such as a vaccine for example, may be "the drop, which to overflow the cup" and to have serious consequences - from mild illness and allergies to severe, incurable diseases and even death. Vaccines not only do not protect efficiently from the diseases, for which they are intended, but on the contrary - they increase the risk of "contagion" and even they themselves can cause (and very often cause) the occurrence of epidemics. If under "prevention" and "treating" is understood reproduction of a disease, then surely they are not desirable.

For everybody should be obviously that the quantity of poisons in the blood as and the degree of resistance are different for each individual. The active anaphylaxis (hypersensitivity) is the alibi or excuse of those who meld "for" vaccines. But that does not change the fact that all vaccines are poisonous, even if they are "clean". Despite of the constant repetition, that they are innocent and harmless, the exact amount of damages/harms, that the immunizations and re-immunizations have caused to humans is not, and will never be known. There are not words that can describe the damages/harms, which the immunizations, vaccines and serums have done and continue to inflict. Closest in meaning is the definition "incomparable vandalism".

After initiation of mass immunizations the standards for diagnosis of an illness were deliberately changed, with purpose the number of sick people to seem less and thus to "prove" the efficacy of vaccines. Officially are not recognized either immediate or deferred in time side effects from vaccines. The lack of obvious immediate reactions after a vaccination does not mean that chronic immunological and/or neurological problems do not occur. Despite the extreme censorship on real results from the immunizations, many experts acknowledge that vaccines often cause severe illnesses and even death: syndrome of sudden infant death, coma, multiple sclerosis, paralysis, autism, epilepsy, diabetes, hepatitis, and others. mental and/or physical disabilities. In developing countries have been used special vaccines for the people, in order to reduce birthrate by causing infertility.

Why the wild, free-living in nature animals do not get sick from the "infectious" diseases, although they are not vaccinated? Because they have better immune system than people and they eat without problem from full with microbes ground and water. And the immune system is maintained very simply - by keeping the laws of the Nature. Any free-living, wild animal eats only food that is pursuant with its anatomical and physiological characteristics. And the food is always raw! Also the animals do not use "medicines" and other narcotics.

5. Fluorine (F). The main elements, necessary for building of bones are calcium, fluorine and vitamin D, but only in raw and fresh foods they are combined in the right combinations with other microelements (vitamins, enzymes, carbohydrates, amino acids, fatty acids etc.), which are necessary for their utilization.

The fluorine, which is recommended to be taken in pure form by water fluoridation, toothpaste or fluoride tablets, to be built strong bones (and most of all teeth), is a pure poison!

Till 1945 the fluorides had been considered for one of the most dangerous environmental pollutants. They are more poisonous than lead and slightly less poisonous than arsenic! The fluorides have been the cause for many lawsuits against industrial production. Fluorine compounds are major waste products in the aluminum industry and in the manufacture of fertilizers. Still in 1850 fluoride emissions from iron and copper industries poisoned people, animals and damaged/harms crops.

In 1944 in Deep Water, New Jercy, occurred a pollution incident from the factories of the company "Dupont", producing thousands tonnes of fluorides in conjunction with the top secret project "Manhattan" - developing of an atomic bomb. Fluorides had been among the main substances in its manufacture. Findings show that the myth about the safety of these compounds at low doses for humans has been created precisely in connection with the development of the atomic bomb. This myth has been created with two main purposes. First - to downplay the legal claims by citizens and so the industry to prevent itself from the payment of huge benefits. Second - not to be given publicity of cases, so that not to be declassified the project. Scientists, who had been participating in it, had been having the task to provide the necessary "evidences" to support this strategy. Because the first gone to law by a worker in that sinister program had not been due to radiation, and for damages/harms, caused by fluorides!

Due to many other such incidents that had caused deaths and damages/harms to health of humans and animals, as and destruction of plants by fluorine compounds, numerous court acts were begun by survivors against the owners of the respective factories. To minimize losses for payment of benefits and to continue production, as without problems to dispose their toxic waste products in the environment, the owners of these industries even have decided to establish their own laboratories with corrupt scientists, whose task has been to "prove" by experiments and researches the harmlessness and even the usefulness for health of certain waste products, such as the fluorine compounds. In practice, were not reported actual results of studies and experiments, and false, favorable results. In order not to state to public the true facts they have used censorship, intimidations, ridicule, revocation of medical rights and other means against professionals, who have tried to state the real facts.

As a result of that, in 1950, after bribery and of political lobbies, Public Health Service (PHS) of U.S.A. formally approved fluoridation. Since then, annually about 450,000 tonnes toxic fluorides have been poured in more than half of the drinking water reservoirs of the U.S.A., Canada, Australia and New Zealand. In such way the industrial giants have got two purposes simultaneously. First - they save money for neutralization and/or safe storage of poisonous waste fluorine compounds, as and for payment of any compensation for pollution and damage/harm of the Nature. Second - they earn from their sale, as they are used for fluoridation of water and toothpastes.

Initially and in most European countries had been applied fluoridation of drinking water, but once it had been discovered that not only it was not useful for health, but also was harmful, it has been prohibited. In Denmark fluoridation of water was prohibited in 1964, in Germany - in 1971, in Sweden and in Netherland - in 1972. In Bulgaria from 1970 to 1971 began the widespread use of fluoride tablets. In the middle of the 80^{-s} of the last century, free fluoride tablets were given to about 500,000 children and students. In 1971 there was a decree of the Council of Ministers with special instruction for artificial fluoridation of drinking water. Fortunately it has not been implemented in practice.

And here are the true facts about "the usefulness and the harmlessness" of fluorides:

- Over the years fluorides are accumulated in bones. The kidneys can eliminate only 50% of their daily intake. One of the consequences of this process is skeletal fluorosis (including dental fluorosis), which makes bones weak and fragile, and also is caused and joint disorders (arthritis).
- Fluorides are cancer-generating. They mainly affect to the genetic material of the cell, as even half of the quantity, which is used for fluoridation of water, significantly damages/harms DNA. Various studies show that they induce and osteosarcoma (bone cancer), cancer of the oral cavity, thyroid cancer, liver cancer, kidney damages/harms.

- Just one millionth of a gram (1 ppm /part per million/), and dose of fluoridation of drinking water is usually higher, inhibits enzyme systems in the cell, causes birth defects in animals and humans, destroys the immune system, violates collagen synthesis and contributes to the calcification of soft tissues, makes worse or causes arthritis.
- In the scientific literature there are evidences, showing that the fluorides cause and delayed replacement of milk teeth with permanent ones. This leads to curvature and dislocation of the teeth in the mouth, which requires putting of braces, splints.
- The fluorides, which are put into drinking water, are contaminated with a variety of other toxic and/or carcinogenic metal compounds with cumulative effect - aluminum, arsenic, radium! So that the liquids, which people intake, are toxic cocktails. All drinks (including so-called "natural juices"), which are made with fluoridated and/or chlorinated water are very harmful for life and health.
- Levels of fluoride in the water between 3 and 11 parts per million directly damage/harm brain, before to damage bones. Bioavailability of aluminum in the body is increased in the presence of fluorine compounds, as in the brain is found a double increase of this toxic metal. It is occurred destruction of nerve cells and also a significantly higher risk of developing of dementia, Alzheimer's disease, impaired motor function, of the intelligence, people become stupid and obedient.
- Fluorides are in the composition of warfare neuroparalytic gas sarin, psychotropic "medications" and sleeping pills, painkillers and pesticides.

6. Radioactive and chemical substances (gases, fertilizers, pesticides, herbicides, insecticides, etc.) in the environment, ultraviolet, X-ray and laser rays.

6.1. Diethylstilbestrol. This is an artificial sexual hormone that is widely used in food industry. It is found that 85% of meat and dairy products contain hazardous residues from it. It (and not phantom viruses and bacteria - as it is claimed by the representatives of the official medicine) is one of the causes for cancer of uterine, of breast and of other reproductive organs, change of sexual orientation and/or premature sexual maturation.

6.2. Nitrosamines. It is scientific proved that nitrosamines cause cancer of the liver, stomach, brain, bladder, kidneys and other organs. They are formed in the body from nitrites and nitrates, chemical preservatives and dyes, which are commonly used today.

6.3. Hexachlorophene. Ingredient in many disinfectants, cosmetics, detergents and cleaners. It causes brain damage/harm and cancer.

7. Paraffin wax (artificial wax). It is produced by crude oil and it forms toxic sludge in the body. That sludge occludes the organism. Often dealers or manufacturers put wax on fruits and vegetables, so that to preserve them longer and they to have a shiny appearance. There isn`t an organ, including the liver, which can process crude oil or petroleum products. So better avoid lustrous fruits and vegetables, or for surer remove their bark - even of those that are commonly eaten. It is unfortunate that they contain many very useful nutrients.

We are creators of our tomorrow day and no need to pay to a "diviner", whether a doctor, a lawyer, a priest or a banker, to tell us what will happen to us tomorrow. Nothing special will happen. The inevitable will occur - we will reap what we have sown.

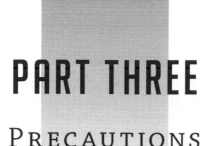

PART THREE
PRECAUTIONS

As it was mentioned earlier, to prevent us from diseases should be kept the natural hygiene of the body. To maintain external cleanliness is clear. And to maintain internal purity must keep the principles of the natural hygiene.

1. First principle - consumption only of foods, which are suitable for the relevant organism.

In the second part are listed facts with details, which indisputably prove that humans are anatomically and physiologically adapted to eat only plant foods, and more precisely - raw and fresh fruits, vegetables, grains and nuts. Besides the harmful (toxic) foods do not consume and the other harmful/poisonous substances, which are mentioned in "Part two".

2. Second principle - nutrition according to the natural cycles of the body.

The physiological cycles of the body have been researched by many scientists, as most of the researches have been the work of Swedish scientist Aare Vaerland, American T.K. Fry and Gay Gear Luke. In short: the ability of the human body to degrade and absorb of food depends on the efficient functioning of three regular daily cycles. These cycles are: digestion (eating and degradation of food), absorption of nutrients and excretion of waste products. Although to some extent these functions take place continuously, each one of them is more intense in certain periods of the day:

- From 1200 hrs to 2000 hrs - digestion (eating and degradation);
- From 2000 hrs to 0400 hrs - absorption of nutrients;
- From 0400 hrs to 1200 hrs - excretion of waste products.

Because for each of these processes is spent much energy, it is very important to eat only from 1200 hrs to 2000 hrs. Otherwise there will not be enough energy for full digestion and assimilation of food, as and for excretion of waste products from it (and from metabolism in general). Exactly the retention of waste products of metabolism, which are toxic, leads to various health problems.

3. Third principle - consumption of foods with high water content (fresh, raw "live" foods).

The word "vegetarian" comes from the Latin word "vegetus", which means "strong, alive."

Human life primarily depends from air, at second place - from water and at third place - from food. The human body consists of 70% pure, distilled water. It needs from 2 to 4 liters of water per day. Water is obtained by drinking of water, other fluids and digestion of food. The best drink for humans and other animals is naturally existing fresh water. It is not harmful, as any other artificial man-made drinks. Drink spring water or mineral water with low mineralization. Especially beware of fluorine (F). It should be below 1.0 mg/l. Do not drink chlorinated water. Chlorine was used during World War I as combat poison gas! It should not be drunk water during or immediately after eating, because it dilutes the gastric juices. Thus is slowed digestion, extra energy is consumed, and food begins to rot and ferment.

From foods, which are suitable for man only fresh, raw fruits and vegetables are with high water content. All other foods are concentrated. Even some food contains a lot of water, its quantity greatly reduces by heat treatment. Moreover, when a food is cooked above 50 degrees Celsius (due to the high temperature and biochemical reactions, which occur) all vitamins, enzymes, trace elements, carbohydrates, amino acids and fatty acids are destroyed or become unusable.

Vitamins are low molecular organic substances, which are necessary in minimum quantities for normal vital activity of humans and animals. About 30 vitamins are known today. They influence (directly or as active ingredients of enzymes, nucleotides) to growth, metabolism, immune function, nervous and endocrine systems, hematopoiesis, coagulation, etc..

Enzymes are molecules that catalyze biochemical processes in the cell. Typical enzymes are proteins or protein complexes, but there are RNA with enzymatic function - so called "ribozymes". Biochemical reactions in the body can be accelerated by the enzymes up to 1 million times.

Once the body is consist from 70% water, must predominate foods with high water content. It is desirable that at least 70% of the food, that is consumed per day, to consist of raw and fresh fruits and vegetables. It is desirable and nuts to be eaten raw, because they also contain essential vitamins, enzymes, carbohydrates, proteins, fats and microelements, which are destroyed by heat treatment. If predators eat heat treated meat, they also will get sick, even though their body is adapted to eat meat - unlike our own.

There are two important reasons why do we need raw and fresh food: nutrition and purification of organism. Naturally containing water in raw, fresh foods is absorbed more easily by the organism itself, because raw food is degraded and absorbed more easily. Thus naturally dissolved vitamins, enzymes, carbohydrates, amino acids, fatty acids and micronutrients by blood reaches every cell of the body. The artificial vitamins and minerals from pharmacies, as any artificial thing, are not fully absorbed by the body and much contaminate kidneys and liver.

The second important task of water is purification (detoxification) of the body from the toxins in it. Heat treated foods are acidifying, i.e. poisonous. They clog your body with poisons; they take much energy for digestion, absorption and excretion of waste products; they cause constipation, obesity, gout, etc.. Some people are thin and do not gain weight, despite they eat too much. This is because some of their glands or organs do not work properly, in result of that the food is not totally degraded and digested, and it is excreted from the body unused. Appetite is big, because the body needs of lacking vitamins, enzymes, trace minerals, amino acids, fatty acids and carbohydrates. Their mistake is that these people tend to consume unhealthy foods and drinks. Sooner or later their glands and/or organs will be completely exhausted.

4. Fourth principle - proper combination of foods.

One of the first scientists, who have dealt with problems about nutrition is Russian Ivan Pavlov. He had researched conditioned reflexes, and particularly in nutrition and in 1902 was printed his book "The work of the digestive glands". I. Pavlov has found that substances, which prevail in different foods cause the release of various gastric juices. For example, when in a food dominate carbohydrates, in the stomach is released alkaline gastric juice, which is necessary for their degradation. When in a food predominate proteins, is released acidic gastric juice. Another eminent scientist, who practiced natural treatment and extensively studied the issue of proper food combining, was american physician Dr. Herbert M. Shelton.

It was already mentioned, that most energy was spent for digestion - up to 80%! People, like all other animals, are not adapted to degrade and assimilate simultaneously more than one type of food. Most people not only eat different foods (most of which generally are not suitable for them), but they eat them simultaneously. This overburdens very much digestive glands and organs, contributes to the accumulation of many harmful waste products, consumes much energy and usually leads to gain of weight.

When simultaneously (or after insufficient time interval) is consumed proteins and carbohydrates, in the stomach are released acidic and alkaline juices, which are neutralized. The body produces new juices, which takes time and energy. The new juices are also neutralized. These processes repeat many times for a long time and they consume much energy. Foods have started to rot and ferment. Such foods release into the body poisonous gases and acids.

In fact, every food contains carbohydrates, proteins and fats, but in most foods predominates only one type substance. Therefore foods are divided into three groups - carbohydrates, proteins and fats, depending on which substance prevails in them. There are a few exceptions - in pulses, for example - soya, beans, lentils. They contain almost the same percentage of carbohydrates and proteins, but even in them is contained a certain quantity of vitamins, enzymes and microelements, which are necessary for full and rapid degradation of that type of food. But despite of that are got gases and abdominal pains, which are evidences for decay and fermentation.

For proper food combining is important not only different foods not to be consumed simultaneously, but also to wait some time between meals. Each type of food is degraded and absorbed for different times. Fruits are degraded and absorbed fastest. Of course they must be fresh and raw! The slowest and most difficult are degraded and absorbed animal products.

Time for digestion (stay in stomach) of the various foods:

- Raw fruits - up to 1 hour;
- Raw vegetables - 2 hours;
- Heat-treated vegetables - 3 hours;
- Raw carbohydrates - 3 hours;
- Heat-treated carbohydrates - 4 hours;
- Raw vegetable proteins - 3 hours;
- Heat-treated vegetable proteins - 4 hours;
- Raw animal proteins - 4 hours;
- Heat-treated animal proteins - 6 hours;
- Improperly combined foods - 8 hours;
- Raw fats - 7 hours;
- Heat-treated fats - up to 10 hours.

Fruits		
Acid	**Semi-acid**	**Sweet**
oranges	apples	bananas
tangerines	pears	grape
grapefruits	peaches	figs
pineapples	apricots	dates
strawberries	cherries	all dried fruits
lemons	plums	water melons
kiwi	grape	melons
sour apples	papaya	
sour grape	mango	

sour cherries	blackberries	
tomatoes	raspberries	
	blueberries	

Leafy green vegetables

lettuce	green onion	zucchini
salads	onion	dock
cabbage	garlic	leeks
cucumbers	okra	spinach
cauliflower	celery	nettles
broccoli	brussels sprouts	parsley
pepper	tinea	sorrel
endive	turnip	eggplant
green dock	green beans	

Carbohydrates (starch)

Starchy proteins	Starchy vegetables	Light-starchy vegetables
coco nuts	potatoes	carrots
pulses - beans, lentils, peas, beans and others	sweet potatoes	beet
grains - wheat, rye, barley, rice, buckwheat, millet, oats and others	Jerusalem artichokes (artichoke)	pumpkin
	corn (maize)	grain sprouted seeds

Proteins

Other vegetable	Nuts	Seeds	Germinated	Animal
soya	acorns	sunflower	soyabean	fresh milk
avocado	almonds	sesame	bean	cheese
olives	hazelnuts	pumpkin seeds	lentils	yellow cheese
mushrooms	walnuts		sunflower	yogurt
	cashew		sesame	any kind of meat

	chicory			eggs
	peanuts			

Fruits are combined badly with leafy green vegetables, carbohydrates and proteins.

Green leafy vegetables are combined well with carbohydrates (starch) and proteins.

Carbohydrates (starches) are combined badly with proteins.

1. Carbohydrates can be combined among them.
2. Do not eat together two or more different proteins.
3. Do not eat acid fruits with sweet ones.
4. It is best to consume honey, dissolved in tea or water. It is combined bad with all foods.
5. Oils and fats are combined well with all foods other than fruits, but should be used in very small quantities, because they delay digestion too much - up to 10 hours.
6. Use spinach rare, and it to be raw.
7. Tomatoes are acidic fruit. They can be combined with carbohydrates and vegetables.
8. Avoid peanuts and peanut butter, because they are hard for digestion.

Sample menu, which is complied with the principles of the Natural hygiene:

- Breakfast - from 0800 hrs to 1100 hrs - must be drunk water, and optionally - herbal tea with honey. If you are hungry, you can eat raw, fresh seasonal fruits or to drink fruit juice, but only freshly squeezed juices from raw, fresh fruits.
- Lunch - from 1200 hrs to 1300 hrs - a salad from raw, fresh seasonal vegetables, wholemeal bread and optionally - soup or dish from vegetables. Do not eat fried foods!
- Dinner - from 1700 hrs to 1900 hrs - a salad of raw, fresh seasonal vegetables (optionally sprinkled with 5-10 g sesame) and up to 50 g of raw, fresh nuts (walnuts, almonds or hazelnuts).

(Note: The intervals of time for each one feeding do not mean that they can or should be used for eating continuously throughout the whole period of time. They are just recommended intervals for nutrition.)

5. Fifth principle - do not overeat!

After overeating digestion is delayed, it is consumed a lot of energy, the digestive glands and organs are overworked and exhausted. Moreover, most people gain weight.

6. Sixth principle - movement.

Life is movement. Movement is health. Health is wealth.

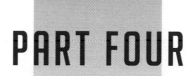

PART FOUR

TREATMENT

Only the Nature can heal. It can not give the treatment (even it wants) to the medical doctors. The human body is a part (and not an exception) from the Nature, and it can self-maintain and self-treat, if are kept the principles of the Natural hygiene. Living human being, like all other living organisms, is designed and operates under the laws of the Nature. The symptoms, by which a disease manifests, are result of self-regulatory and protective functions of the body, and they should be supported with fasting and good external hygiene.

The only proper, efficient, reasonable, fast and safe treatment for diseases, developed due to poor natural hygiene, is fasting and, if it is possible, to avoid harmful emotions (anger, worry, fear), which also take energy, which is necessary for digestion and absorption of foods, as and excretion of waste products from the body. During fasting is given opportunity to the body to clean and to heal by itself. The diseases are treated successfully, as even damaged/harmed glands and organs are recovered, but if they are not completely exhausted or damaged/harmed. Very often the representatives of official medicine say that some disease is autoimmune or congenital (inherited) and incurable, just because they do not know the true cause for the disease and can not cure it. (Unfortunately, genetic/congenital diseases are not healed with anything.)

During a fasting is saved a lot of energy (up to 80%), which is used for digestion and absorption of food. The saved energy is spent for degradation, neutralization and excretion of accumulated poisons in the body. Moreover, new toxic substances do not enter into the body, which additionally poison it, and it is not spent energy for neutralization and excretion of them. The immune system is strengthened. It is given a rest of the organs and glands. It is changed to internal (endogenous) feeding, the body begins to degrade tumors (if any), thrombus (if any), kidney stones and gall bladder (if any), crystals in the joints (arthritis) - if any, fatty formations (including fatty plaques in blood vessels), and other poisons that have been accumulated in the body. The weight is reduced (with about 1 kg/day) and the body is rejuvenated. The wounds heal.

To keep the achieved results is very important after a fasting to be done a proper breakfasting and to be kept natural way of life!

1. Types of fasting.

There are two types of fasting: fasting and starving (the phase after fasting).

Fasting is two types: strict and soft.

During the strict form of fasting is intaken only water. Maybe someone has heard or read for "Urine-therapy." This perverted and abnormal form of fasting, during which is not consumed anything else (usually) own urine, has many disadvantages. First - a man to adapt itself psychologically to drink only that disgusting-looking, disgusting-smelling and perhaps even more disgusting on taste liquid. Second - any urine, as a waste product, is extremely poisonous, and any subsequent excretion logically becomes more concentrated and more toxic. Third - highly acidic liquid. Perhaps the only positive effect is loss of weight. If there is any healing effect, it occurs very slowly.

During the soft form of fasting is consumed a limited quantity (up to 1 kg/day) of raw and fresh (not dried concentrated) fruits (or fresh squeezed juices from raw, fresh fruits) or raw, fresh vegetables (or fresh juices from raw, fresh vegetables).

2. Advantages of soft form of fasting with raw (fresh) fruits, herbal tea and honey:

2.1. It is not required a hospital treatment and supervision by a physician. (Except for certain serious chronic diseases that are dependent on "medicines" - diabetes, high blood pressure, epilepsy, etc.. They require daily measurements of certain parameters and gradual reduction of "medicines.")

2.2. Fruits are digested and absorbed quickest by the body and it is spent least energy, in compare with other foods. At the same time they provide energy and many nutrients for the body. The raw, fresh fruits contain:

- Carbohydrates in the form of fructose. Unlike concentrated white sugar and white flour, the raw, fresh fruits contain all the necessary enzymes, vitamins and microelements, which are necessary for the rapid degradation of fructose to glucose. So, fruits are suitable even for treatment of diabetes!
- Easily digestible and absorbable proteins.
- Easily digestible and absorbable fats.
- Lots of vitamins, enzymes, minerals, fibers and water.

2.3. The raw, fresh fruits contain pure water that is closest in composition to the protoplasmic fluid in a living cell, and which is most easily absorbed by the body.

2.4. Even acidic fresh fruits in the body react alkaline, as it is very important for slightly standing of the acid crisis. During changing to the endogenous feeding, the toxic waste products are being increased, and they are acidic. By fruits body receives fruit acids that are unstable and rapidly are oxidized to carbonic acid (H_2CO_3), which dissociates and the formed CO_2 is released during respiration by the lungs. Hydrogen atoms are connected with oxygen in the air and is formed water. In this way the alkaline ingredients of fruits neutralize acids, obtained from waste products in the body. Thus are ensured normal conditions for the flow of biochemical processes and is accelerated the excretion of toxins.

2.5. Natural vitamins and enzymes, contained in raw, fresh fruits are quickly and easily absorbed. They act as catalysts for biochemical processes.

2.6. The activity of the digestive system does not stop completely (as it is in the case of the strict form of fasting). During of slow mastication of the fruits they are mixing well with saliva. In this way is done pre-made degradation of carbohydrates by ptyalin enzyme, contained in the alkaline saliva. Staying of fruits in stomach is halved. The faster passage of fruits in the gut does not create conditions for fermentation. Furthermore, the mastication reduces and suppresses an eventual sense of hunger by central mechanism (via the hypothalamus), which is highly expressed during fasting only with water. As slower is mastication of fruits as greater is peristaltic of bowels. With the increase of peristaltic waves is being accelerated the excreting of harmful toxic materials with feces. Cellulose components in fruits, which are contained in them, also help for these processes. Enemas are unnecessary.

2.7. During the strict form of fasting is recommended the patient to lie, in order not to spend energy for motion. Energy is required for degradation and excretion of toxic wastes. During immobilization is being decreased muscle tone. During fasting with fruits is recommended walks in the fresh air and light exercises, which maintain the tone of muscles, despite of reducing of weight. By movements is assisted and excretion of toxins through the skin during sweating.

2.8. Eating of 2-3 teaspoons pure honey. It is concentrated and valuable food that contains carbohydrates (as many sugars), water, minerals, nitrogen compounds, proteins, enzymes, organic acids, vitamins, colourants, royal jelly, aromatic compounds, biogenic stimulators, plant antibiotics and etc.. Intaking small quantities of honey prevents the fasting man to reach to hypoglycemic conditions. Sugars (fructose and glucose) are valuable not only because of the energy that they provide, but also for their healing effect. The absorption of fructose through the cell membrane is not related to the presence of insulin, which is very important in the treatment of diabetes and also in the treatment of liver, heart, metabolism, etc.. Glucose and fructose during fasting help for regulating of nerve activity, expand blood vessels, improve nutrition of the heart muscle, intensive urination, improve metabolism, regulate heart rate, lower blood pressure. The action of biochemical processes is not affected.

3. Practice of softened form of fasting with fresh fruits, herbal tea with honey and water.

3.1. During fasting must not be consumed anything else but raw and fresh seasonal fruits, herbal tea with honey and water! If somebody suffers from a serious illness, such as diabetes, epilepsy, hypertension and others, for which he must drink "medicines", compulsory the fasting must be done under the supervision of a doctor, who has sufficient theoretical and practical training not only in fasting and natural-based nutrition, but also and in official medicine. The doctor every day performs the necessary examinations and tests, and he can determine when and how to begin to reduce the "medicines" and when to stop fasting.

May be used only raw, fresh seasonal fruits: up to 1 kg/day acidic or semi-acidic fruits or up to 2kg/day watermelons. It is desirable to consume only one type of fruits, and they must be chewed slowly and well. Avoid sweet and dried fruits, because they are concentrated and very caloric, thus reduces the therapeutic effect and reduction of overweight.

3.2. Determination of duration of fastings and the intervals between them.

Depending on the disease should be done different in number and duration fastings. In acute forms of diseases usually is enough one short fasting. In chronic diseases and/or too much contaminated with poisons organism is needed to apply more prolonged fasting, and sometimes and several fastings. (E.g.: in arthritis, spurs, large tumors etc..) Duration of fasting depends on the type and extent of disease, depending on the physical and mental tolerance of the patient - from 1 to 25 days and sometimes more.

In the beginning of fasting may occur so-called "crisis of fasting": increased appetite, weakness, exasperation, tension, headache, nausea, changes in blood pressure, pain in the affected areas in ulcers, arthritis, etc.. These crisis are as more severe and longer as the body is more damaged/harmed and there are more poisons in it, but usually crisis are no longer than 5 days. The symptoms of crisis of fasting are as more pronounced as more toxic and sick is organism, because the blood is saturated with toxic wastes.

At mild suffering of a fasting, it may continue for at least 14-15 days. At severe suffering of fasting sometimes is needed it to continue from 1-2 to 3-4 days, which to be repeated after 8-10 to 12-15 days, during which nutrition must be natural-based - according to the principles of the natural hygiene.

After a short fasting (from 3 to 7-8 days) and 5-day breakfasting, the intermediate interval must be respectively from 8 to 20 days. After a long fasting (from 10-15 to 20-25 days) and 10-day breakfasting, the interval of natural-based nutrition must be respectively from 4-5 to 7-8 weeks!

It is desirable, if it is possible, a fasting to be done according to the following scheme:

At 0800 hrs - and during all day you can drink low mineralized or spring water, but must there are intervals of at least 1 hour before and after eating of fruits, so as not to dilute the gastric juices.

At 0900 hrs - a cup of herbal tea with a teaspoon pure honey or water as you want. Honey should not be heated above 40 degrees Celsius!

At 1000 hrs – a portion of fresh fruits (300 g).

At 1200 hrs - a cup of herbal tea with a teaspoon pure honey or water as you want.

At 1400 hrs – a portion of fresh fruits (300 g).

At 1600 hrs - a cup of herbal tea with a teaspoon pure honey or water as you want.

At 1800 hrs – a portion of fresh fruits (300 g).

3.3. The interruption of a fasting must be compulsory by a special breakfasting!

During fasting the digestive system is with reduced functions and it must be gradually adjusted to its normal work. Therefore, the transition between fasting and normal nutrition must be done by special breakfasting. Otherwise, cured diseases can be regenerated, and even they can get worse. There are instances with people, who had done an inappropriate breakfasting, and for that then have been occurred severe crisis, coma and even death. Therefore it is very important a proper breakfasting to be done with a certain duration, which depends on the duration of fasting.

During breakfasting, as well as fasting, is very important not to use toxic substances for the human body, including legal narcotics - coffee, non-herbal tea, alcohol, soft drinks, cigarettes and "medicines" (except for the vital at the moment "medicines"). It is also very important gradually to increase the types and quantities of foods, but not to overeat!

After a fasting from 3 to 10 days is enough breakfasting of 5 days, and after a fasting from 11 to 25 days must be done 10-day breakfasting.

SCHEME OF 5-DAY BREAKFASTING
(After 3 to 10-day fasting)

First day

At 0800 hrs - a cup of herbal tea with a teaspoon pure honey or water as you want. Honey should not be heated above 40 degrees Celsius!

Throughout the day you can drink low mineralized or spring water, but must there are intervals of at least 1 hour before and after eating of food, so as not to dilute the gastric juices.

At 0900 hrs – a portion of fresh, raw fruits (300 g).

At 1000 hrs – a portion of fresh, raw fruits (300 g).

At 1200 hrs - about 150 g of fresh seasonal vegetables.

At 1500 hrs - you may drink water.

At 1600 hrs - a cup of herbal tea with a teaspoon pure honey or water as you want.

At 1800 hrs – a portion of 200 g fresh, raw seasonal vegetables.

Second day

At 0800 hrs - a cup of herbal tea with a teaspoon pure honey or water as you want. Honey should not be heated above 40 degrees Celsius!

Throughout the day you can drink low mineralized or spring water, but must there are intervals of at least 1 hour before and after eating of food, so as not to dilute the gastric juices.

At 0900 hrs – a portion of fresh, raw fruits (300 g).

At 1000 hrs – a portion of fresh, raw fruits (300 g).

At 1200 hrs - 300 g fresh seasonal vegetables and a small boiled potato without salt.

At 1500 hrs - you may drink water.

At 1600 hrs - a cup of herbal tea with a teaspoon pure honey or water as you want.

At 1800 hrs - 300 g salad of fresh, raw seasonal vegetables and 300 ml vegetable soup of potato, carrot, cabbage - no spices.

Third day

At 0800 hrs - a cup of herbal tea with a teaspoon pure honey or water as you want. Honey should not be heated above 40 degrees Celsius!

Throughout the day you can drink low mineralized or spring water, but must there are intervals of at least 1 hour before and after eating of food, so as not to dilute the gastric juices.

At 0900 hrs – a portion of fresh, raw fruits (300 g).

At 1000 hrs – a portion of fresh, raw fruits (300 g).

At 1200 hrs - 300 g salad of seasonal fresh, raw vegetables and fresh oats (a small coffee-cup of oat is soaked in three such cups of water for at least one hour).

At 1800 hrs - 300 g salad of fresh, raw seasonal vegetables, a portion of steamed vegetables (potatoes or green beans) and a slice of bread. For the first time to salad you may add and a pinch of salt and few drops of oil.

Fourth day

At 0800 hrs - a cup of herbal tea with a teaspoon pure honey or water as you want. Honey should not be heated above 40 degrees Celsius!

Throughout the day you can drink low mineralized or spring water, but must there are intervals of at least 1 hour before and after eating of food, so as not to dilute the gastric juices.

At 0900 hrs – a portion of fresh, raw fruits (300 g).

At 1000 hrs – a portion of fresh, raw fruits (300 g).

At 1200 hrs - 300 g salad of fresh seasonal vegetables, 1-2 slices of bread and a few unsalted olives.

At 1800 hrs - 300 g salad of fresh, raw vegetables and pre desalinated cheese - as the matchbox.

Fifth day

At 0800 hrs - a cup of herbal tea with a teaspoon pure honey or water as you want. Honey should not be heated above 40 degrees Celsius!

Throughout the day you can drink low mineralized or spring water, but must there are intervals of at least 1 hour before and after eating of food, so as not to dilute the gastric juices.

At 0900 hrs – a portion of fresh, raw fruits (300 g).

At 1000 hrs – a portion of fresh, raw fruits (300 g).

At 1200 hrs - 300 g salad of fresh, raw seasonal vegetables, 3-4 slices of bread and a portion of boiled white beans (without roux and hot/chilli spices!).

At 1800 hrs - 300 g salad of fresh, raw seasonal vegetables and 30-40 grams of raw nuts (almonds, walnuts or hazelnuts).

If you plan do not eat more dairy products, instead of them you can use raw nuts!

SCHEME OF 10-DAY BREAKFASTING
(After more than 10-day fasting)

First day

At 0800 hrs - a cup of herbal tea with a teaspoon pure honey or water as you want. Honey should not be heated above 40 degrees Celsius!

Throughout the day you can drink low mineralized or spring water, but must there are intervals of at least 1 hour before and after eating of food, so as not to dilute the gastric juices.

At 0900 hrs – a portion of fresh, raw fruits (300 g).

At 1000 hrs – a portion of fresh, raw fruits (300 g).

At 1200 hrs - about 150 g of fresh, raw seasonal vegetables.

At 1500 hrs - you may drink water.

At 1600 hrs - a cup of herbal tea with a teaspoon pure honey or water as you want.

At 1800 hrs - 200 g fresh, raw seasonal vegetables.

Second day

At 0800 hrs - a cup of herbal tea with a teaspoon pure honey or water as you want. Honey should not be heated above 40 degrees Celsius!

Throughout the day you can drink low mineralized or spring water, but must there are intervals of at least 1 hour before and after eating of food, so as not to dilute the gastric juices.

At 0900 hrs – a portion of fresh, raw fruits (300 g).

At 1000 hrs – a portion of fresh, raw fruits (300 g).

At 1200 hrs - 300 g fresh seasonal vegetables and a small boiled potato without salt.

At 1500 hrs - you may drink water.

At 1600 hrs - a cup of herbal tea with a teaspoon pure honey or water as you want.

At 1800 hrs - 300 g fresh, raw seasonal vegetables and a small boiled potato without salt.

Third day

At 0800 hrs - a cup of herbal tea with a teaspoon pure honey or water as you want. Honey should not be heated above 40 degrees Celsius!

Throughout the day you can drink low mineralized or spring water, but must there are intervals of at least 1 hour before and after eating of food, so as not to dilute the gastric juices.

At 0900 hrs – a portion of fresh, raw fruits (300 g).

At 1000 hrs – a portion of fresh, raw fruits (300 g).

At 1200 hrs - 300 g salad of fresh seasonal vegetables and a large boiled potato without salt.

At 1800 hrs - 300 g salad of fresh, raw seasonal vegetables and 300 ml vegetable soup of potato, carrot, cabbage - no spices.

Fourth day

At 0800 hrs - a cup of herbal tea with a teaspoon pure honey or water as you want. Honey should not be heated above 40 degrees Celsius!

Throughout the day you can drink low mineralized or spring water, but must there are intervals of at least 1 hour before and after eating of food, so as not to dilute the gastric juices.

At 0900 hrs – a portion of fresh, raw fruits (300 g).

At 1000 hrs – a portion of fresh, raw fruits (300 g).

At 1200 hrs - 300 g salad of fresh, raw seasonal vegetables and two large boiled potatoes without salt.

At 1800 hrs - 300 g salad of fresh, raw seasonal vegetables and 300 ml vegetable soup of potato, carrot, cabbage - no spices.

Fifth day

At 0800 hrs - a cup of herbal tea with a teaspoon pure honey or water as you want. Honey should not be heated above 40 degrees Celsius!

Throughout the day you can drink low mineralized or spring water, but must there are intervals of at least 1 hour before and after eating of food, so as not to dilute the gastric juices.

At 0900 hrs – a portion of fresh, raw fruits (300 g).

At 1000 hrs – a portion of fresh, raw fruits (300 g).

At 1200 hrs - 300 g salad of fresh, raw seasonal vegetables and a slice of bread.

At 1800 hrs - 300 g salad of fresh, raw seasonal vegetables and 300 ml vegetable soup of potato, carrot, cabbage. For the first time to salad and soup, add a pinch of salt and few drops of oil.

Sixth day

At 0800 hrs - a cup of herbal tea with a teaspoon pure honey or water as you want. Honey should not be heated above 40 degrees Celsius!

Throughout the day you can drink low mineralized or spring water, but must there are intervals of at least 1 hour before and after eating of food, so as not to dilute the gastric juices.

At 0900 hrs – a portion of fresh, raw fruits (300 g).

At 1000 hrs – a portion of fresh, raw fruits (300 g).

At 1200 hrs - 300 g salad of fresh, raw seasonal vegetables and raw oats (a small coffee-cup of oats is soaked in three such cups of water for at least one hour).

At 1800 hrs - 300 g salad of fresh, raw seasonal vegetables, a portion steamed vegetables (potatoes or green beans) and 1-2 slices of bread.

Seventh day

At 0800 hrs - a cup of herbal tea with a teaspoon pure honey or water as you want. Honey should not be heated above 40 degrees Celsius!

Throughout the day you can drink low mineralized or spring water, but must there are intervals of at least 1 hour before and after eating of food, so as not to dilute the gastric juices.

At 0900 hrs – a portion of fresh, raw fruits (300 g).

At 1000 hrs – a portion of fresh, raw fruits (300 g).

At 1200 hrs - 300 g salad of fresh, raw seasonal vegetables, a few slices of bread and portion of boiled peas.

At 1800 hrs - 300 g salad of fresh, raw vegetables and seasonal pre desalinated cheese – as matchbox.

Eighth day

At 0800 hrs - a cup of herbal tea with a teaspoon pure honey or water as you want. Honey should not be heated above 40 degrees Celsius!

Throughout the day you can drink low mineralized or spring water, but must there are intervals of at least 1 hour before and after eating of food, so as not to dilute the gastric juices.

At 0900 hrs – a portion of fresh, raw fruits (300 g).

At 1000 hrs – a portion of fresh, raw fruits (300 g).

At 1200 hrs - 300 g salad of fresh, raw seasonal vegetables, a few slices of bread and a portion of lens (without roux and hot spices!).

At 1800 hrs - 300 g salad of fresh, raw seasonal vegetables and 30-40 grams of raw nuts (almonds, walnuts or hazelnuts).

Ninth day

At 0800 hrs - a cup of herbal tea with a teaspoon pure honey or water as you want. Honey should not be heated above 40 degrees Celsius!

Throughout the day you can drink low mineralized or spring water, but must there are intervals of at least 1 hour before and after eating of food, so as not to dilute the gastric juices.

At 0900 hrs – a portion of fresh, raw fruits (300 g).

At 1000 hrs – a portion of fresh, raw fruits (300 g).

At 1200 hrs - 300 g salad of fresh, raw seasonal vegetables, a few slices of bread and a portion of rice with vegetables (without roux and hot spices!).

At 1800 hrs - 300 g salad of fresh, raw seasonal vegetables and 200 g yogurt.

Tenth day

At 0800 hrs - a cup of herbal tea with a teaspoon pure honey or water as you want. Honey should not be heated above 40 degrees Celsius!

Throughout the day you can drink low mineralized or spring water, but must there are intervals of at least 1 hour before and after eating of food, so as not to dilute the gastric juices.

At 0900 hrs – a portion of fresh, raw fruits (300 g).

At 1000 hrs – a portion of fresh, raw fruits (300 g).

At 1200 hrs - 300 g salad of fresh, raw seasonal vegetables, a few slices of bread and a portion of white beans (without roux and hot spices!).

At 1800 hrs - 300 g salad of fresh, raw seasonal vegetables and 50-60 grams of raw nuts (almonds, walnuts or hazelnuts).

If you plan do not eat more dairy products, instead of them you can use raw nuts!

To keep the results, achieved after fasting, must be done correct breakfasting, and then to eat natural-based - in accordance with the principles of the natural hygiene, as and to keep a natural way of life - according to the principles of natural lifestyle!

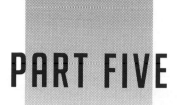

PART FIVE

THE TRUTH ABOUT THE "INCURABLE" DISEASES

Indeed, official medicine can not cure any disease, because either doctors do not know the true causes for diseases, or they do not want to treat diseases, because they are financially interested from that. Here are some of the most often occurring or announced by the official medicine for "incurable" diseases.

1. AIDS - the fraud of the twentieth century.

AIDS dictionary:

- AIDS - syndrome of acquired immune deficiency;
- HIV - human immunodeficiency virus;
- Retrovirus - a virus that cannot reproduce itself and to exist alone, and it multiplies by cell division and can exist only in it;
- AIDS test - a test that detects antibodies to HIV (as the test sample is diluted 400 times!), but not and the virus itself;
- HIV-positive - a positive test for AIDS;
- A virus carrier - who is supposed to be living with HIV, having been HIV-positive;
- Sick of AIDS - a virus carrier, who developed symptoms of at least one of the 30 AIDS-determining illnesses.

Leukocytes	Main target or function
Neutrophils	Bacteria, fungi.
Eosinophils	Large parasites, allergies.
Basophils	Release histamine, in inflammation.
Lymphocytes	B cells: secrete antibodies, antigen presentation. T cells: - T CD4 + - activates and regulates the function of T and B cells. Controller of the immune system; - CD8 + T cytotoxic cells - sick/tumor cells; - Гδ T cell, NK cell: sick/tumor cells.
Monocytes	Precursor of macrophages.
Macrophages	Phagocytosis of cellular debris and parogens, antigen presentation.
Dendritic cells	Antigen presentation.

Leukocytes is general term of all white (not containing hemoglobin) cells. Leukocytes in the blood are divided into three groups: granulocytes, monocytes and lymphocytes. The three groups of cells have a protective function. The main function of leukocytes is phagocytosis, which is implemented by neutrophils, having a role of macrophages and monocytes. Granulocytes in turn unify three different by structural features and functions cells - neutrophils, eosinophils and basophils. Lymphocytes immunologically and functionally are divided into two main types - B and T, which are morphologically unidentifiable. Monocytes in the blood now are considered as a single cell line without subtypes. In peripheral blood establishes metamyelocytes, segment-nuclear and stick-nuclear cells. Single metamyelocytes normally only are found in newborns, and segment-nuclear and stick-nuclear cells - at any age, with a predominance of segment-nuclear granulocytes.

The reasons for the excogitation and dissemination of the false theory about AIDS (that it is a contagious disease, that it is caused by HIV, etc.) are:

- doctors, pharmacists and their political lobbies legally to steal money from state budgets, in the form of subsidies amounting to hundreds of milliards of dollars a year for "researches and development of vaccines and "medicines" against HIV";
- further damages/harms to health with vaccines and "medicines" against HIV-positive or sick from AIDS people, as ones are earned money by every sale of vaccines and "medicines" and by "treatment" with them, and second time - by further "treatment" of induced chronic diseases;
- the representatives of official medicine do not to admit, that they have completely failed in curing of diseases, and they have killed and were continuing to kill millions with their poisonous vaccines and "medicines";
- intimidation and panic among people by "infecting" with HIV, to limit the indiscriminate and/or unprotected sexual contacts (to limit promiscuity and fertility in the world), as well as to reduce the number of addicts and homosexuals. (These intentions are really good.)

And what is the truth about AIDS? When the facts speak and "gods" (ignorant or corrupt "experts") and other brazen liars (media) must keep silent!

1. In 1984, Dr. Robert Gallo at a press conference stated that he had discovered a HIV, which caused AIDS. Before to do this statement in the literature had not been published any evidences, also the theory had not been offered to the scientific community, so that to be discussed and to be proved, which was a standard practice! The allegation was stated as firmly established fact, based only on assumptions, coincidences and correlations. Later the false theory has been imposed across the world again without any evidences, but only on the basis of international agreement. Since then in the scientific literature there has been no one evidence that HIV caused AIDS, as at the same time has been imposed very strict censorship about the real causes for AIDS, as and for cancer!
2. The retrovirus HIV has never been found and isolated! The AIDS test actually detects antibodies, and not the virus itself. The presence of

antibodies is not compulsory an indication for presence of a virus, nor for a disease of the immune system, and just the opposite - indicates that the immune system has responded. Especially during the test for HIV is clear that the antibodies, which are searched, are found in everybody. Some people have them in high concentrations, while others - in low, but only if are found very high levels of antibodies, the test is defined as a positive. Therefore, when is made test for AIDS, the sample, which is taken for "discovery" of HIV, is diluted 400 times! Otherwise all samples will be positive! When the antibodies are many, it means that the immune system has detected an increased quantity of some antigens in the body.

3. In cases of advanced AIDS (even in people, who are already dying with such a diagnosis) is extremely difficult to "detect" HIV (i.e. - a certain quantity of antibodies), and at least at 50% of cases they are not detected at all (i.e. - there are antibodies, but their number is below the determined abstract limit).

4. According to Dr. Gallo AIDS virus destroys T-cells, and thus the immune system. In fact such a thing never occurs. HIV is a retrovirus, and as such it can not reproduce independently. Its existence depends on the life of the cell, in which it is located, i.e. it can live and multiply, when the cell is alive and is dividing. If the virus destroys the host cell, it would mean to suicide and the "epidemic" would be over before it has started!

5. T-cells multiply 500 times faster than retroviruses (such as HIV). T-cells recognize, attack and destroy diseased cells in the body. (T-cells are a type of lymphocytes, and they are one of the three main groups of leukocytes /white blood cells - protective cells of the immune system/. Other two groups are granulocytes and monocytes).

6. More than 20 years of intensive researches have found that retroviruses (such as HIV) did not kill cells, and just the opposite - they made them to multiply faster. So that they were the subject of attention from side of researchers, working on the causes for cancer. It is impossible the same virus in some cases to "destroy" cells, as in pneumonia, while in others to make them to multiply - as in Kaposi's sarcoma!

7. Viruses are found in many types of bacteria and simple life forms like bacteria. Viruses are constant elements (components) of different cells, living together in a single cell type, as the bacteria into the cells of animals and humans assist for transfer of oxygen (i.e. they help the mitochondria)

or as the bacteria in all plants assist for producing of oxygen (i.e. they help the chloroplasts). This is called "endo simbiosis" (mutually beneficial cooperation), which occurs in the process of combining different cell types and structures. In fact, scientifically proven role of viruses in the higher complex interactions of cells is to assist, support and in no way to destroy!

8. If somebody has positive test for HIV and at the same time is sick from one of 30 or more well-known diseases, such as pneumonia, dementia, Kaposi's sarcoma, tuberculosis, lymphoma and others, he is diagnosed as ill from "AIDS". AIDS is not a disease, and damage/harm of the immune system!

The true causes for AIDS (i.e. reducing the strength of the immune system) are poisoning of the body due to: improper nutrition, intake of harmful (toxic) substances for the organism and harmful emotions; poor diet or systematic malnutrition - lack of vitamins, enzymes, microelements, carbohydrates, amino acids, fatty acids, etc.. (That is why there are most patients, sick from AIDS, in the U.S.A /where people eat very unhealthy and are used many narcotics - narcotics are very strong poisons for the immune system and for body as a whole/ and in poor, underdeveloped countries /e.g. in African countries, where people eat improperly and/or poor).

The "treatment", which the official medicine applies, is like for all diseases: additional poisoning of the body, while is being tried to destroy "pathogenic" microorganisms with the poisonous "medicines". For example, in the early 90^{-s} patients were "treated" with Zidovudine (AZT), Dideoxyinosine (ddI), Dideoxycytidine (ddC). All these "medicines" had been originally designed to kill cancer cells by chemotherapy, and as they destroyed any cells, which they reached, of course they caused and all side effects during such "therapy" - hair loss, muscle degeneration, anemia, nausea, vomiting, etc.. AZT has even been suspended from use, because it had been found that it was too toxic even for cancer patients in final stage of their disease! Side effects of AZT are listed on the instruction: lymphomas (cancer), hepatitis, dementia, mania (madness), epileptic seizures, anxiety, anemia, leukopenia, impotence, severe nausea, chest pain, insomnia, ataxia, depression, muscle atrophy, etc..

Treatment. The only proper, efficient, reasonable, fast and safe treatment of AIDS (and for all diseases) is to eliminate the causes (stopping to intake of poisonous substances for humans). When body is intoxicated - detoxication by fasting, proper breakfasting, natural-based nutrition and lifestyle (according to the principles of natural hygiene), and in deficiency of vitamins, enzymes, micro elements, carbohydrates, amino acids or fatty acids (due to poor diet or systematic malnutrition) - natural-based nutrition and lifestyle.

2. Cancer (tumors, cysts, myomas).

2.1.Causes. According to official medicine, causes for most types of cancer (and the type is defined from the part of the body, which is affected) are viruses or bacteria. Official medicine divides it into "benign" (in less damage/formation, which is not increased and spread into the body) and "malignant".

The real causes for cancer are: poisoning of the body (see "Toxic/harmful substances for the human body"), concentration and (bio)chemical actions of poisons on the cells, tissues or organs; lack of nutrients or oxygen to cells; ultraviolet, X-ray, laser or radioactive radiation; mechanical irritation. Cancer is the last stage of a chronic degenerative disease.

Why then are continued to spread informations that the causes for cancer are not known and incorrectly is assumed, and sometimes allegedly, that again viruses and bacteria are guilty? Why do governments spend tens of milliards of dollars annually for researches for the causes of cancer and for developing of "medicines" and vaccines for its "treatment"? Because the official medicine is a selfish and a monopolistic system, searching financial gain that operates on the principle: "more diseases - more profits". Therefore, the absolute elimination of diseases, including cancer, contrary to its financial interests. The illnesses are a large business, business for hundreds of milliards of dollars annually. Cancer and AIDS are diseases that provide some of the biggest revenue for medical-pharmaceutical mafia.

Cancer may be:

- a lump, which may be a hard fatty or protein formation (e.g. mastitis - a lump in the breast) from accumulated toxic waste products;
- swollen lymph node due to the concentration of poisons in it;

- damaged/harmed or dead cells of the body, due to: their intoxication; lack of oxygen or nutrients to them; radioactive, ultraviolet, X-ray or laser rays.
- peel (thickening) of the surface of an ulcer (wound).

To stop the absorption of poisonous substances directly through a wound by the blood from wounded blood vessels, and also to prevent internal bleeding, the body strives to close the ulcer (as any wound) with thickening (bark), which doctors call "cancer" and they cut it. If this thickening is formed on pyloric (stomach outlet to the duodenum), it gradually is closed, and foods and drinks begin to be vomited. If thickening is on the exit, entrance or anywhere in the colon, doctors also call it "cancer", and cut it. But this does not eliminate the causes!

The lymphatic system is base of the defense (immune) system. It produces lymphocytes - one of the three main groups of white blood cells in the body. The whole body is covered with glands/nodes that purify the lymph fluid and they are connected by lymph links between them. You can touch those lymph nodes, which are located on shallow under the skin - at sides of the neck, under the chin, at armpits and near to groins. **Tonsils** are the largest lymph nodes in the body. They represent a protective barrier against antigens and is extremely improper their removal (as and of any other lymph nodes) in the inflammation/swelling. Often "preventively" (not to "spread" the cancer) are removed whole glands, tissues or organs (for example - one or both the breasts), in which has been found a lump. When the quantity of accumulated in the body poisons is greater than their removal, some lymph node, in which poisons are too much, may swell. If the amount of toxins continue to rise, they are transferred to nearby lymph node. (So-called "metastasis").

2.2. "Healing" methods of the official medicine.

- Chemotherapy (see for AIDS).
- Radiation therapy - also harmful for the body irradiations by laser rays to kill cancer cells (but are damaged/harmed and healthy cells around them).

- Surgically - removal of swollen lymph nodes, break of the links between them, removing of lumps (from solidified waste products or dead cells) - removal of the consequences, but not and of the causes! It is more spectacularly (and profitably) to make surgeries instead to teach people how to live in order to avoid chronic diseases and surgeries.

Cancer cells are damaged/harmed or dead cells of the body, due to: their intoxication; lack of oxygen or nutrients to them; radioactive, ultraviolet, X-ray or laser rays. Therefore, only the ignorant, irresponsible or criminal "doctors" can apply these methods of "treatment"! These are extremely harmful, ineffective and vandal methods, actually not of treatment, and of additional poisoning and damage/harm of the body or a mutilation of it during unnecessary removal (because of ignorance) very often of whole glands, tissues or organs (e.g. during breast cancer) and often causing of death. Why are then they applied? Because only they are officially accredited and approved for "treatment", and only for them are given huge amounts from government budgets (i.e. taxes of the people) to the "hospitals" for "treatment" of cancer.

2.3. Precautions. They are as for all acquired diseases - respect for the laws of the Nature. Natural way of life - natural-based nutrition, avoidance of toxic/harmful substances for the body, movement.

2.4. Treatment. If you are diagnosed with "cancer", first do not worry. Treatment depends only on you, if the phase of illness is not final. The only proper, efficient, reasonable, fast and safe treatment is eliminate of the causes (stopping to intake of poisonous substances for humans), fasting, proper breakfasting and natural-based lifestyle. Allow to the representatives of the official medicine to use their murderous methods for "treatment" for themselves and for people who can not or do not want to stop their harmful habits. Surgery is necessary only in case of full blockage of the digestive, urinary, respiratory or cardiovascular system.

3. Leukemia.

Literally translated from Greek means "white blood". It is a disease with origin from bone marrow (but it is not the cause for disease!), which is characterized with the production of "pathological" white blood cells, also called "parablasts".

The blood cells (leukocytes, erythrocytes, platelets) are produced by bone marrow. Before the mature and functional cells to enter into the bloodstream, they undergo development, as they are passing through different stages. White blood cells originate from precursor cells, which by division go through a series of intermediate forms, to reach mature leukocytes, capable for performing of their functions - protection against foreign agents, found into the body (sick/dead cells, parasites, toxins, etc.). Unlike the solid tumors, which form a tumor somewhere in the body, leukemia are diseases that occur as a combination of malignant cells, circulating in the bloodstream. Leukaemia is a pathological condition, in which there is an abnormal maturation of white blood cells - they can not reach its final stage of development and fall into blood immature, in that way they can not perform their functions.

▬ 3.1. "Treatment" by methods of the official medicine.

Leukaemia is "cured" by conventional medicine by various methods: by "medicaments" (chemotherapy), radiotherapy or, in some cases - by a bone marrow transplant. Different "medicines" are used intravenously, orally, in cerebrospinal fluid by lumbar puncture, intramuscular, subcutaneous and they only additional poison the body!

▬ 3.2. Treatment. Due to the poisoning of the body and harm of functions of bone marrow, the only proper, rational, efficient, fast and safe treatment is detoxification (cleansing) of the body by fasting, proper breakfasting and natural-based lifestyle (stopping to intake of poisonous substances for humans).

4. Gout, disc disease, spurs, arthritis (including the private case - disease of Bechterev), (pyelo)nephritis, stones around the teeth, in the kidneys and in the gall.

Gout is caused by increased acidity in the blood due to excessive toxic substances in the body. Strong (urinary) acids are formed during improper food combining, when are consumed foods from animal origin, heat -treated foods (especially fried foods!), sugar and confectionery, bakery and pasta made from white flour, hot, sour, salty, alcohol, "medicines", coffee, not-herbal tea and others narcotics, soft drinks, artificial colours, flavours, preservatives, food additives, etc.. When the acids reach to the kidneys, gallbladder, joints or spine, they begin to irritate their mucous, causing pain and damages. It is possible to retain water in the body, to dilute harmful acids. When acids are retained for long time in the blood, they begin to precipitate and crystallize in the joints, spine, kidney or gallbladder, and are formed solid formations. Crystals are enlarging, and spine and joints are swelling (spurs, disc disease, arthritis) or are being formed kidney stones or in the gall. Tophus is formed, when are eaten acidic-forming substances, mostly fried foods and heat-treated fats.

Treatment. The only proper, reasonable, effective, safe and quick treatment is eliminate of the causes (stopping to intake of poisonous substances for the human body), fasting, proper breakfasting and natural-based lifestyle (including and natural-based nutrition).

5. Epilepsy.

From Greek it means "attack". Also it is known as "Morbus Sacer" (from Latin it means "sacred disease") and is one of the most common neurological diseases, characterized by recurrent swoons. Today one of every hundred people in the world suffers from epilepsy. People, suffering from epilepsy are called "epileptics".

5.1. Types of swoons. Epileptic seizures are divided into many subspecies, but the main division is in two types. These are focal and partial. During the focal a person may experience cramp, severe headache, hallucinations, feeling scared, anxiety. Often the symptoms stop so far, but the patient's condition may deteriorate and he to start to get partial swoons. The partial are divided into two subspecies: petit mal (from French, meaning "little sickness") and grand mal (from French - "big disease").

When a epileptic gets a type of swoon "petit mal", he just is freezing at place and he is non-contact for a few seconds, then he "wakes up" and continues as if nothing has happened. If the swoon is weaker, the patient may not even freeze, and just to continue to do his work, without even to exhibit any symptoms, that he has got a swoon. In both the cases, the patient is little likely to remember whether he has had a swoon or not. About 80% of epileptics get swoons type "petit mal", which are easily treated.

When a epileptic gets a type of swoon "grand mal" and he "is freezing" after a few seconds he is starting to shake (or he is falling on the ground - if he is standing), his mouth is being filled with foam, but sometimes it happens and eyes to turn inwards and/or to release on a small need. This swoon lasts longer than "petit mal" and after that the patient simply falls asleep, and when he wakes up he does not remember anything.

5.2. Causes. Epilepsy is caused due to damage/harm of part of the brain due to:

- choking the baby during birth and lack of oxygen to the brain;
- in people with cancer, the possibility of getting epilepsy is greater; the same goes for people, who have suffered a severe injury of head;
- use of vaccines, "medicines" and other narcotics;
- an unfavorable combination of genes.

5.3. What are seizures caused from?

In patients with epilepsy there is a field in the brain (so-called "hearth"), which causes the swoons. As the nerve connections in the brain are very complex and intertwined, when the epileptic "hearth" "sends a signal," it confuses these links, and for that in those parts of the brain, controlling different parts of our body, confuses are occurred. Sometimes, before getting of an epileptic seizure, the patient gets hallucinations, he does not feel well, etc. According to some, when one gets an epileptic seizure, then the brain "resets" (it "switches off and switches on" again).

5.4. Treatment. If the part of the brain is not completely damaged/harmed, the best treatment is fasting, proper breakfasting and natural-based lifestyle (stopping to intake of poisonous substances for humans). "Treatment" by "medicines" and herbs only reduces somewhat the grade of seizures, but does not remove the causes, i.e. if the cause is a tumor or action of poisons, which inhibit the affected control center.

6. Diabetes.

During the intake of refined sugar and sugar products, artificial sweeteners, bakery and pasta from white flour the quantity of blood sugar is increasing rapidly. And to decrease quickly the level of blood sugar, is overworked the pancreas. It produces the hormone insulin, which is necessary for digesting of sugar. On the other hand some vaccines, "medicines", alcohol or other narcotics, as and a systemic psychological stress harm/frazzle directly the pancreas or exhaust it.

Treatment. If the pancreas is not completely damaged/harmed, the only proper, reasonable, effective, safe and quick treatment is eliminate of the causes (stopping of negative emotions and of intake of poisonous substances for the human body), fasting (especially in overweight), proper breakfasting and natural way of life (including and natural-based nutrition).

7. Hypoglycemia.

During systemic low level of blood sugar (due to producing of much insulin after intake of refined sugar and sugar products, artificial sweeteners, bread and pasta, made from white flour), during systemic stress situations or during use of vaccines, "medicines", alcohol or other narcotics is secreted a significant quantity of adrenaline. It is one of the hormones, which are produced by the adrenal glands. It increases metabolism of carbohydrates, to increase the level of blood sugar. If the adrenal glands are exhausted or with reduced functions (Addisons disease), the level of blood sugar remains low, even the pancreas does not produce insulin at a time.

Treatment. The only proper, reasonable, effective, safe and quick treatment is eliminate of the causes (stopping of negative emotions and of intake of poisonous substances for the human body), fasting (especially in overweight), proper breakfasting and natural-based lifestyle (including and natural-based nutrition).

8. Hepatitis.

This is inflammation of the liver. The name comes from Greek - hepar (ἧπαρ - liver) and the suffix-itis, (ίτις - inflammation).

The first clinical symptoms of acute hepatitis vary from asymptomatic (no visible signs) to fatigue, yellowing of the skin and/or eyes, nausea, vomiting, dizziness or diarrhea. Hepatitis is a non specific term, used to define inflammation of the liver. It is diagnosed by a blood test that shows an increase of liver enzymes.

The causes for hepatitis are not viruses or bacteria (as is claimed by the representatives of the official medicine), and damage/harm of liver from poisons, including the so-called "medicines".

Treatment. If the liver is not completely damaged/harmed, the only proper, reasonable, effective, safe and quick treatment is eliminate of the causes (stopping to intake of poisonous substances for the human body), fasting (especially in overweight), proper breakfasting and natural way of life (including and natural-based nutrition).

9. Allergies, "venereal" and skin diseases (dermatitis, psoriasis, periodontitis, eczema, herpes, fungus, hay fever etc.).

Causes. Again, according to the official medicine for these diseases are guilty microorganisms. The truth is that when the quantity of toxins in the body is large, it strives to exude them and by the skin and/or mucous membrane, and they can be irritated additionally and by external irritants - dust, pollen, light, etc.. Where toxins are most concentrated, sores and wounds are caused, which are occurred more quickly during poor external hygiene and scratching or friction/rubbing. "Treatment" by ointments or antibiotics does not help, and can only harm!

Treatment. The only proper, reasonable, effective, safe and quick treatment is eliminate of the causes (stopping to intake of poisonous substances for the human body), fasting (especially in overweight), proper breakfasting and natural-based lifestyle (including and natural-based nutrition).

10. Overweight.

It is caused from impaired metabolism due to bad habits, but mostly during non-compliance of principles of natural hygiene. Most affecting are non-compliance of the natural cycles of the body, improper combination of foods, use of heat-treated foods, foods from animal origin, sugar and confectionery, bakery and pasta made from white flour, overeating.

Treatment. The only proper, reasonable, effective, safe and quick treatment is eliminate of the causes (stopping to intake of poisonous substances for the human body), fasting, proper breakfasting and natural-based lifestyle (including and natural-based nutrition).

11. Hypertension, arteriosclerosis and dementia.

The causes for persistently high blood pressure are: narrowed blood vessels by fatty plaques, polluted kidneys or use of any narcotics.

Fatty plaques are obtained by eating of heat-treated foods (especially fried foods), animal products, hydrogenated and hydrolyzed fats. They are the cause and for **arteriosclerosis and dementia**. Biochemical reactions that occur in fats, when they are being heated, make them difficult degradable and difficult assimilable. They are superimposed on the walls of the cells, as gradually become visible (by a naked eye) overlays in various tissues and organs, including blood vessels. And overlays in stomach and intestines obstruct to the absorption of the nutrients.

The kidneys are most polluted by consumption of harmful substances for the human body.

"Treatment" by "medicines", which is used by the official medicine, is harmful and ineffective, because the "medicines" have dangerous side effects and do not remove the causes for the diseases.

Treatment. The only proper, reasonable, effective, safe and quick treatment is eliminate of the causes (stopping to intake of poisonous substances for the human body), fasting (especially in overweight), proper breakfasting and natural-based lifestyle (including and natural-based nutrition). If those diseases are left untreated, that may cause bleeding in various places on the body, including heart attack (infarct) or brain hemorrhage. Normal blood pressure is 120/80 +/-10.

12. Low blood pressure and anemia.

The cause for the constant low blood pressure and anemia is the reduced quantity of hemoglobin, leading to reduced blood volume, due to poisoning of the body, improper or inadequate nutrition. Hemoglobin is the iron-containing pigment in red blood cells (RBCs), whose main function in the body is the transport of oxygen and carbon dioxide. From foods that are suitable for people most iron contain raw leafy vegetables, beet and beans.

Treatment. The only proper, reasonable, effective, safe and quick treatment is eliminate of the causes (stopping to intake of poisonous substances for the human body), fasting (especially in overweight), proper breakfasting and natural-based lifestyle (including and natural-based nutrition). "Doctors" recommend to be eaten foods from animal origin (meat especially), because there the concentration of iron (an essential element for building of hemoglobin) is biggest. But this is only true for raw, fresh animal products, because after a heat treatment is destroyed the majority of iron in them! But even if the animal products are eaten raw, they are sufficiently harmful for the human body. It is the best to drink at least 0.5 liters/day juice from raw, fresh carrots and beets in 1/1 ratio.

13. Multiple sclerosis.

(Encephalomyelitis disseminata, also known as "multiple sclerosis", abbreviated MS.) According to the "doctors" (representatives of official medicine) it is an autoimmune, infectious, neurodegenerative chronic disease with unknown etiology and possible genetic predisposition. Therefore, those "doctors" can not cure it!

Causes. Multiple sclerosis affects the fatty myelin sheath of axons of the human main and spinal brain. Because of entry of toxic substances in the brain are occurred hyperplasia (expansions) of the connective tissue of nerves. This causes demyelination (destruction of nerve sheaths) and formation of lesions (damages) in the brain, leading to a wide spectrum of signs and symptoms. The main symptoms are: weakness, strong convulsive movements, lack of coordination of limbs, delirium, coupled by hallucinations, affecting of speech, uncontrollable rapid eye movements, convulsive tremor (which disappears completely during a rest or a sleep), sudden loss of vision of one eye, double vision, strange feelings of tingling and numbness in various parts of the limbs and body, problems with the rectum and bladder.

Treatment. The only proper, reasonable, effective, safe and quick treatment is eliminate of the causes (stopping to intake of poisonous substances for the human body), fasting (especially in overweight), proper breakfasting and natural-based lifestyle (including and natural-based nutrition).

14. Tuberculosis.

It is a chronic-occurring, specific, inflammatory disease that mainly affects the lungs but can affect the central nervous system, lymph vessels, digestive system, bones, joints and even skin. Official medicine believed that the tuberculosis is caused by microorganisms and can not cure it. The real causes are poisoning of the body (mostly by animal products) or systematic malnutrition.

Treatment. The only proper, reasonable, effective, safe and quick treatment is eliminate of the causes (stopping to intake of poisonous substances for the human body), fasting (especially in overweight), proper breakfasting and natural-based lifestyle (including and natural-based nutrition).

15. Rheum, (bronchial) asthma, (bronchitis)pneumonia, pleurisy, sinusitis, meningitis, purulent tonsillitis, diphtheria, scarlet fever, mumps, smallpox (variola), varicella (chickenpox), measles and rubella.

According to official medicine the causes again are viruses and bacteria, but the real cause is poisoning of the body, especially by foods from animal origin. From waste products from foods from animal origin is formed mucus, which initially is excreted from the nose (**rheum**). If the quantity of toxins is too much, mucus begins to excrete and by the tonsils (**purulent tonsillitis, scarlet fever** - white overlays on the tonsils, mainly from waste products from milk and dairy products, **diphtheria** - gray overlays on the tonsils, mainly from waste products from meat and meat products or **mumps** - inflammation and swelling of salivary glands around the ears - mainly from waste products from milk and dairy products).

If the causes are not eliminated, may develop chronic diseases - **(bronchial) asthma, (bronchitis)pneumonia, pleurisy, sinusitis, meningitis or tuberculosis** (caused due to retention of toxic waste products in the relevant organs). In most children the immune system is not enough strong (mostly due to poor diet /because of their harmful habits of nutrition/ and additional poisoning by "medicines" and numerous mandatory vaccines), therefore can be developed so-called "typical childhood diseases": **smallpox, chickenpox,**

measles and rubella. Specific for these diseases is the appearance of small or large rashes on the skin, which are caused when the body is attempting to eliminate poisons and by the skin. They are not infectious, although it is claimed by the official medicine. "Infectious" are just people's habits, including the harmful ones!

Treatment. The only proper, reasonable, effective, safe and quick treatment is eliminate of the causes (stopping to intake of poisonous substances for the human body), fasting (especially in overweight), proper breakfasting and natural-based lifestyle (including and natural-based nutrition).

16. Gastritis, colitis, Crohn's disease and ulcer.

The official medicine claims that and they are caused by microbes. The truth is that they are caused from mechanical (not well chewed food), and mostly from chemical (acid) irritation of the stomach, duodenum or intestines. Strong acids are formed after consumption of foods from animal origin, improper combined foods, heat-treated foods (especially fried foods!), sugar and confectionery, bakery and pasta made from white flour, hot, sour, salty, alcohol, coffee, not-herbal tea, "medicines" and other narcotics, soft drinks, artificial colours, flavours, preservatives, food additives, etc..

All poisonous substances for human organism (except concentrated alkalis, such as caustic soda, for example) cause strong acids, which initially cause irritation of the mucosal of stomach or duodenum (**gastritis**), and if the bad habits are not stopped and the causes are not eliminated, is formed a wound (**an ulcer**) on a mucosal. During improper food combining, use of foods from animal origin or heat-treated foods are occurred constipation, fermentation and rotting of foods and waste products from them in the large intestine. The strong acids, which are formed in that case, cause inflammation of its mucosa (**colitis**). If the bad habits are not stopped and the causes are not eliminated, is formed a wound of its mucosa (**ulcer**). If irritation persists, are formed and other ulcers.

To stop the absorption of poisonous substances directly through a wound by the blood from wounded blood vessels, and also to prevent internal bleeding, the body strives to close the ulcer (as any wound) with thickening (bark), which doctors call "**cancer**" and they cut it. If this thickening is formed on pyloric (stomach outlet to the duodenum), it gradually is closed, and foods and drinks begin to be vomited. If thickening is on the exit, entrance or anywhere in the colon, doctors also call it "**cancer**", and cut it. But this does not eliminate the causes!

Treatment. The only proper, reasonable, effective, safe and quick treatment is eliminate of the causes (stopping to intake of poisonous substances for the human body), fasting (especially in overweight), proper breakfasting and natural-based lifestyle (including and natural-based nutrition).

17. Osteoporosis (porous bones) and tooth decay (caries).

When are consumed poisonous substances, in the body is increased blood acidity. Strong acids are formed after consumption of foods from animal origin, improper combined foods, heat-treated foods (especially fried foods!), sugar and confectionery, bakery and pasta made from white flour, hot, sour, salty, alcohol, coffee, not-herbal tea, "medicines" and other narcotics, soft drinks, artificial colours, flavours, preservatives, food additives, etc.. To neutralize the acids, the body takes calcium from bones, which is needed for the formation of carbonate compounds (alkalis).

Treatment. The only proper, reasonable, effective, safe and quick treatment is eliminate of the causes (stopping to intake of poisonous substances for humans), natural lifestyle (including and natural-based nutrition). When a man has overweight, it is necessary before this to be done fasting and proper breakfasting to improve the overall health condition and to reduce the burden on the bones.

18. Migraine.

The cause for periodical or continuous severe headache may be high blood pressure, brain tumor, sinusitis, total poisoning of the body or a mental tension.

Treatment. The only proper, reasonable, effective, safe and quick treatment is eliminate of the causes (stopping to intake of poisonous substances for the human body), fasting (especially in overweight), proper breakfasting and natural-based lifestyle (including and natural-based nutrition).

19. Infertility, impotence, frigidity, menstrual problems or at a pregnancy.

The official medicine again is powerless! Due to poisoning of the body, it may be harmed functions of genitals, it can become blocking of fallopian tubes or infringement of content and/or structure of the cervical mucus, it may be harmed functions of testicles and ovaries. Also may occur functional and/or anatomical changes and of other parts of the reproductive system (including formation of tumors, myomas or cysts; menstrual problems or at a pregnancy).

There are many documented cases of successfully cured infertility of men and women, and also of impotence and frigidity menstrual problems or at a pregnancy by fasting (especially in overweight), proper breakfasting and natural-based lifestyle (including and natural-based nutrition).

20. Mental (psychiatric) diseases.

Most often they are caused from vaccines, "medicines" and other narcotics. If the brain is not completely damaged/harmed, many of these diseases could be cured by fasting, proper breakfasting and natural-based lifestyle (including and natural-based nutrition). Back in the 60^{-s} of last century in Soviet Union were cured and mental illnesses by fasting in a clinic, managed by Professor MD Yuriy Nikolaev.

21. Glaucoma.

Irreversible damage of the optic nerve, because of increased intraocular pressure due to poisoning of the body from: improper diet; use of narcotics, including and of psychostimulants, antidepressants, contraceptives and other "medicines". Risk group are also people with hypertensive, diabetic, overweight. The damage of the optic nerve can lead to partial or total loss of vision.

Treatment. If the optic nerve is not completely destroyed, the only proper, reasonable, effective, safe and quick treatment is eliminate of the causes (stopping to intake of poisonous substances for the human body), fasting (especially in overweight), proper breakfasting and natural-based lifestyle (including and natural-based nutrition).

If something is not treated by fasting, it cannot be cured by anything!

22. Cataract.

Cataract is a pathological condition, in which occurs darkening of a lens, in result of which is distorted vision. Representatives of the official medicine "cure" it only surgically (i.e. by the butcher`s method, because they do not know the causes for that disease) and it is consists in removing of the damaged, dark lens and fitting of a new one.

The cause for cataract is accumulation of toxic substances in the eye lens, which form crystals.

Treatment. The only proper, reasonable, effective, harmless, but not so quick treatment is eliminate of the causes (stopping to intake of poisonous substances for the human body), fasting, proper breakfasting and natural-based lifestyle (including and natural-based nutrition).

23. Acute and chronic appendicitis.

This is inflammation of appendicitis/appendix due to retention of waste products in it, because their quantity has been increased in the guts. Appendix is located strategically place between small and large intestine. It releases highly active substance, which serves to neutralize the poisonous waste products, which can irritate the lining of the colon. After all processes of the metabolism are done and from food is extracted everything necessary for the organism, the waste products are kept in the colon before their excretion from the body.

"Treatment" by tradditional way, used by the official medicine includes the use of antibiotics (to kill "guilty harmful microbes"), and if the inflammation is continuing, is proceeded to surgical removal of the appendix, because according to doctors it is "unnecessary"! The same they think and for tonsils!

Treatment. The only proper, reasonable, effective, safe and quick treatment is eliminate of the causes (stopping to intake of poisonous substances for the human body), fasting (especially in overweight), proper breakfasting and natural-based lifestyle (including and natural-based nutrition).

24. Fever ("cold" or "flu").

Fever is a natural reaction of the body, when there is too much accumulation of toxic substances above the point of tolerance, and at the same time there isn`t enough energy for their neutralization and excretion. Then is raised the body temperature, to accelerate the neutralization and excretion of harmful waste products. The temperature acts as a catalyst in those processes. Temperature is an indicator of illness of the body. It is controlled by the hypothalamus.

Representatives of the official medicine ("doctors") often call the fever "cold" or "flu". For the "first sickness" they blame the cold, and for the "second one" - microbes (usually viruses). The truth is that in winter or when it is cold people get sick more often, because the body always distributes the energy consumption with priority for the various processes, and when is cold it spends more energy to maintain the body temperature. Therefore, if the quantity of toxins in the body is close to the point of tolerance, any additional poison or lack of energy for neutralization and excretion of waste products, leads to a protective reaction of the body or so-called "morbid" condition, which is actually a toxic crisis. And whether it is true that fever is caused by viruses, and why "doctors" have decided to call it "flu" (no matter whether it is "winter", "spring," "summer," "autumn," "swine" "bird," "sheep", etc..)!? (See "The truth about avian flu (H5N1), vaccines and AIDS".)

Due to the "guilty" viruses "doctors" prescribe additional poisons - vaccines and "medicines" (antibiotics), which in the best case eliminate symptoms/ consequences (pain, fever), but slow down the healing, because very often they stop and excretion of the toxic waste products.

Treatment. The only proper, reasonable, effective, safe and quick treatment is eliminate of the causes (stopping to intake of poisonous substances for the human body), fasting (especially in overweight), proper breakfasting and natural-based lifestyle (including and natural-based nutrition).

25. Varicose veins.

Veins are vessels, in which blood moves to the heart. Unlike arteries, veins do not have their muscle fibers. The unidirectional flow of blood in them is supported by venous flaps and by contraction of surrounding muscles. The flaps help the blood not to return due to the high hydrostatic pressure.

Most often varicose veins appear on legs and on the lower part of the colon (rectum) and anus. Cause for varicose veins in the legs is the high pressure in them due to: overweight, high blood pressure or long motionless standing at one place (in standing or sitting position). Over time the walls of the veins are expanded and may tear, causing bleeding.

Hemorrhoids are enlarged veins in the lower bowel (rectum) and anus. The cause is the high pressure in them due to: overweight, high blood pressure, constipation (due to: overeating; improper food combining; consumption of animal products, heat-treated foods, hot/chilli, sour, salty, white flour products, refined sugar and other poisonous substances for the human body, which cause acids, fermentation and decay), sedentary lifestyle, tightness of the anus and rectum due to physical or mental stress.

The most serious complication is formation of blood clots in varicose veins. They cause severe disorder of function of the surrounding tissues and organs. The condition can be complicated by occurring of venous gangrene or haemorrhagic necrosis in the acute phase, which may lead to necessity for removal of the damaged/harmed tissues and organs. If a clot breaks away, it can clog a narrow blood vessel and to cause pulmonary embolism, heart attack (infarct) or brain hemorrhage (insult).

Treatment. The only proper, reasonable, effective, safe and quick treatment is eliminate of the causes (stopping to intake of poisonous substances for the human body), fasting (especially in overweight), proper breakfasting and natural-based lifestyle (including and natural-based nutrition).

26. Parkinson's disease.

Symptoms are: tremor (most often) of the extremities, muscle stiffness, slow movements and others, due to damage/harm from intoxication of nerve centers in the brain that control the relevant muscles.

Treatment. The only proper, reasonable, effective, safe and quick treatment is eliminate of the causes (stopping to intake of poisonous substances for

❖94❖

the human body), fasting (especially in overweight), proper breakfasting and natural-based lifestyle (including and natural-based nutrition).

Whether the disease can be fully cured depends on the stage of disability of the brain.

27. An enlarged prostate, cystitis.

The prostate is a subsidiary organ of the male reproductive system. It is located below the bladder, around its neck. The prostate gland secretes a fluid that is mixed with sperm, when it reaches the urethra. Because of its location around the urethra, when the prostate is being increased, it obstructs the movement of urine, which leads to retention of part of it in the bladder. The retention of urine causes irritation, inflammation and erosion of the urethra and bladder neck or bladder inflammation (**cystitis**). All these effects cause painful need for micturition and pain when urinating. The retention of urine causes additional poisoning of the body and even can cause death.

The causes for enlarged prostate are unknown for official medicine. The causes for enlarged prostate are: poisoning of the body, mostly due to not natural-based eating, overeating, use of "medicines", coffee, alcohol, tobacco and other harmful substances, as and excessive sexual excitement.

Treatment. The official medicine uses surgical method for removing of the prostate or part of it, injections for shrinking and other "treatments", which only lead to temporary relief. Furthermore, the surgical method leads to death in 25% of cases and to complications in the remaining 75%, due to failure to make a perfect drainage.

The only proper, reasonable, effective, safe and quick treatment is eliminate of the causes (stopping to intake of poisonous substances for the human body), fasting (especially in overweight), proper breakfasting and natural-based lifestyle (including and natural-based nutrition).

In conclusion, as people pay attention to their health, when they are already severely, chronically ill, the treatment is often difficult, long or impossible. Therefore, it is the best to prevent a disease, rather than to wait to get sick, and then resort to treatment.

BIBLIOGRAPHY
(USED LITERATURE)

"Toxemia explained" – Dr. John H. Tilden

"Fasting – a friend and a medicine" - Lydia Kovacheva

"Fasting can save your life" - Dr. Herbert Shelton

"The science and fine art of fasting" - Dr. Herbert Shelton

"The science and fine art of food and nutrition" - Dr. Herbert Shelton

"Natural hygiene" - Dr. Herbert Shelton

"Hygienic system" - Dr. Herbert Shelton

"Fasting for health" - Prof. M.D. Yuriy Nikolaev

"The miracle of fasting" - Dr. Paul Bragg

"Healthy lifestyle" - Dr. Paul Bragg

"Healing fresh/raw vegetable and fruit juices" - Dr. Norman Walker

"Natural way to vibrant health" - Dr. Norman Walker

"Become younger" - Dr. Norman Walker

"Pure & simple natural weight control" - Dr. Norman Walker

"The medical millennium" - Dr. William Hay

"How to be always well?" - Dr. William Hay

"A new health era" - Dr. William Hay

"Health via food" - Dr. William Hay

"Fit for life" - Harvey and Marilyn Diamond

"Fit for life - a new beginning" - Harvey Diamond

"Stop hair loss" - Dr. Paavo Airola

"How to keep us slim, healthy and young with juice fasting" - Dr. Paavo Airola

"Are you confused?" - Dr. Paavo Airola

"How to get well - handbook of natural healing" - Dr. Paavo Airola

"There is a cure for arthritis" - Dr. Paavo Airola

"Cancer - causes, prevention and treatment" - Dr. Paavo Airola

"Censured for curing of cancer" - Dr. Max Gerson

"Inventing the AIDS virus" - Prof. Dr. Peter Duesberg

"Infectious AIDS - have we been misled?" - Prof. Dr. Peter Duesberg

"Deadly deception - the proof that sex and HIV absolutely do not cause AIDS" – Dr. Robert Willner

"How to raise a healthy child...inspite of your doctor?" - Docent M.D. Robert Mendelsohn

"Confessions of a medical heretic" – Docent M.D. Robert Mendelsohn

"Never ill" - Dr. Robert Jackson

"Food is your best medicine" - Dr. Henry Bieler

"The global conspiracy against the health" - Dr. Atanas Galabov

"The Medical mafia - how to get out of it alive and take back our health and wealth?" –Dr. Guylaine Lanctot

"Medical retribution" ("Expropriation of health") - Ivan Illich

"The drug story" - Morris Bealle

"Vaccines - are they really safe and effective?" - Neil Miller

"Vaccines – the genocide of the third millennium" - Dr. Stefan Lanka and Dr. Karl Krafeld

"Living with death and dying" - Dr. Elizabeth Kubler-Ross

"The dangers of GMOs - a quick guide on "Monsanto" & toxic GMOs in our food supply" – Joey Cardillo

"What doctors don't tell you?" (The truth about the dangers of modern medicine) - Lynne McTaggart